INSULIN RESISTANCE

A Clinical Handbook

To Alison, Jonathan and Robert

Insulin Resistance

A Clinical Handbook

Andrew J. Krentz MD, FRCP

Consultant in Diabetes and Endocrinology
Honorary Senior Lecturer in Medicine
Southampton University Hospitals, UK

Blackwell
Science

© 2002 by Blackwell Science Ltd
a Blackwell Publishing Company
Editorial Offices:
Osney Mead, Oxford OX2 0EL, UK
    Tel: +44 (0)1865 206206
Blackwell Science, Inc., 350 Main Street, Malden, MA 02148-5018, USA
    Tel: +1 781 388 8250
Blackwell Science Asia Pty, 550 Swanston Street, Carlton, Victoria 3053,
Australia
    Tel: +61 (0)3 9347 0300
Blackwell Wissenschafts Verlag, Kurfürstendamm 57, 10707 Berlin,
Germany
    Tel: +49 (0)30 32 79 060

First published 2002 by Blackwell Science Ltd

Library of Congress Cataloging-in-Publication Data
Krentz, Andrew J.
    Insulin resistance : a clinical handbook / Andrew J. Krentz.
        p. cm.
    Includes bibliographical references and index.
    ISBN 0-632-05662-2
    1. Insulin resistance—Handbooks, manuals, etc.
    I. Title. [DNLM: 1. Insulin Resistance. WK 820 K92i 2000]
    RC662.4 .K74 2000
    616.4'6207—dc21
                                                        00-037824

ISBN 0-632-05662-2

A catalogue record for this title is available from the British Library

Set in 9/12 Galliard by Graphicraft Limited, Hong Kong

For further information on Blackwell Science, visit our website:
www.blackwell-science.com

Contents

Preface

Previously a sub-speciality interest among diabetologists, insulin resistance has become relevant to clinicians in many specialties—cardiology and reproductive medicine being two prominent examples. This book aims to provide an introduction to insulin resistance for clinicians who do not have an extensive knowledge of metabolic medicine.

From my perspective as a clinical investigator I have sought to emphasize the clinical implications of current knowledge. I have also pointed out continuing uncertainties, of which there is no shortage! The complex interactions between genes and environment, for example, caution against optimism for an early resolution of some fundamental issues.

I have tried to produce a balanced overview that sets the scene for future developments. Early in this new millennium it seems reasonable to express cautious optimism about future therapeutic prospects. However, alarming rates of obesity, type 2 diabetes and the metabolic syndrome emphasize the need for more effective interventions.

Comments are welcome at **a.j.krentz@soton.ac.uk.**

A.J. Krentz
Southampton, Spring 2002

About the author

Dr Krentz qualified from the University of Birmingham, UK and trained in diabetes and endocrinology in Birmingham and Albuquerque, USA. His doctoral thesis focused on the regulation of intermediary metabolism in insulin-resistant states. Dr Krentz is an active member of the European Group for the study of Insulin Resistance (EGIR) and contributes to the editorial boards of several scientific journals.

Acknowledgements

My thanks go to Andrew Robinson, Gina Almond and Alison Brown of Blackwell Science for advice, encouragement and practical support. Mentors who have my gratitude include Malcolm Nattrass, David Schade and Cliff Bailey. Peter Hale, Dev Singh, Penny Clark, Janet Smith and others made invaluable contributions to the metabolic studies cited from the General Hospital, Birmingham, UK. Malcolm Nattrass and Peter Hale developed the low-dose incremental infusion technique discussed in section 1.5.3.

1 Pathophysiology of insulin resistance

1.1 Introduction

Insulin resistance, a reduced biological effect of endogenous or exogenous insulin, is a common biochemical entity that is associated, either directly or indirectly, with a range of non-communicable human diseases. Insulin resistance may be entirely genetically determined (as in rare syndromes of severe insulin resistance) or acquired, either during intrauterine development or during adolescence and adult life. Relative insulin resistance is also a transient feature of a number of physiological states in humans.

The clinical impact of insulin resistance ranges from subclinical hyperinsulinaemia to major life-limiting disturbances of carbohydrate and lipid metabolism. The main clinical concern derives from the association between impaired insulin action and the development of vascular disease. Microvascular disease is a complication of type 2 diabetes mellitus, in which insulin resistance is a prominent feature. Atherosclerotic macrovascular disease, on the other hand, has a more complex association with insulin resistance that extends beyond hyperglycaemia.

Insulin resistance and human disease

Decades of experimental research have established insulin resistance as a major component in the aetiology of type 2 diabetes, by far the most common form of diabetes worldwide. In type 2 diabetes, insulin resistance is regarded as either the primary metabolic defect or as an important modifier of glycaemia.

Type 2 diabetes carries a well-recognized risk of organ failure resulting from damage to the microvasculature of the retina, kidney and peripheral nerves. However, it is the two- to fivefold increased risk of atherosclerotic disease of the coronary, cerebrovascular and peripheral circulations

Margin notes:

Insulin resistance denotes a reduced biological effect of insulin

Insulin resistance is a transient feature of some physiological states

Insulin resistance is a major component in the aetiology of type 2 diabetes that is responsible for the deaths of 70% or more of patients. Lesser degrees of glucose intolerance share some of the increased risk of atheroma associated with type 2 diabetes. Such individuals can generally be shown to have evidence of insulin resistance. Insulin resistance has also come to be regarded as a risk factor for atherosclerotic cardiovascular disease in the non-diabetic population. This recognition derives, in large part, from Gerald Reaven's (1988) Banting Lecture to the American Diabetes Association. In his presentation, Reaven drew strands of epidemiological and experimental research together to postulate that resistance to insulin-stimulated glucose disposal is the fundamental defect responsible for the clustering of a number of risk factors for atheromatous cardiovascular disease (Syndrome X).

Insulin resistance is implicated in the aetiology of coronary heart disease

Intense research activity has expanded the role for insulin resistance in human disease. Today the notion of insulin resistance as a pathological entity pervades many areas of clinical medicine from diabetes through gynaecology to cardiology, touching on other specialties such as neurology, nephrology and hepatology. Insulin resistance is also of relevance to clinicians treating obesity, lipid disorders, hypertension, trauma, burn injury or the acquired immuno deficiency syndrome (AIDS). In addition, maternal and fetal under-nutrition has emerged as a public health concern with the formulation of the Barker hypothesis of intrauterine metabolic programming. The range of disorders in which insulin resistance is recognized is extensive and is still growing.

Insulin resistance is a feature of many human disorders

The global incidence and prevalence of insulin resistance are increasing rapidly, reflecting alterations in diet and physical activity which are implicated in the increasing burden of obesity and diabetes. Fortunately, greater understanding of the aetiology and pathophysiology of insulin resistance has led to important recent advances in drug therapy. There has also been a resurgence in interest in well-established drugs—notably the biguanides. Thus, at the start of the new millennium, the scene is set for more effective therapeutic intervention.

The global prevalence of insulin resistance is increasing rapidly

Insulin resistance—a pathophysiological enigma

Despite considerable progress, fundamental questions concerning the causes and clinical impact of insulin resistance remain. What, for example, is the molecular basis of the most commonly encountered forms of insulin resistance? How do we define and measure insulin action *in vivo*? Exactly what role does insulin resistance have in the aetiology and progression of common disorders such as type 2 diabetes? How can insulin resistance be avoided or effectively countered? Does insulin resistance directly result in atherosclerosis or might it be a permissive factor or epiphenomenon? Are the molecular defects responsible for insulin resistance a consequence of genetic, environmental or intrauterine factors? Although hyperinsulinaemia and other features of the insulin resistance syndrome can be identified in a proportion of apparently healthy individuals, the prevalence of insulin resistance in the general population is unknown. In part, this uncertainty reflects:

• Difficulties in defining insulin resistance.
• The practical problems of quantifying insulin action.

These difficulties continue to impede therapeutic intervention.

1.2 Normal physiology

In healthy individuals, plasma glucose concentrations are tightly contolled by a complex and integrated system, the principal hormonal regulator of which is insulin. Disturbances of this system may lead either to hypoglycaemia or, more commonly, chronic hyperglycaemia, i.e. glucose intolerance or diabetes. Multiple interrelated homeostatic mechanisms exist to maintain glucose concentrations within the physiological range.

1.2.1 Hormonal regulation of metabolism

Metabolic effects of insulin

Insulin (Fig. 1.1) is the principal anabolic hormone of the body, exerting actions on intermediary metabolism, ion

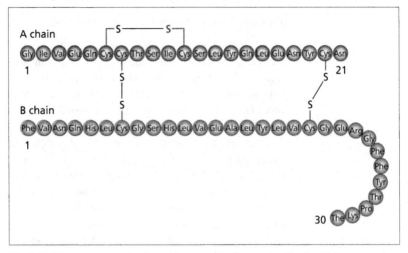

Fig. 1.1 Primary structure (amino acid sequence) of human insulin. Insulin has a complex tertiary structure with a hydrophobic core and a hydrophilic surface.

Table 1.1 Main physiological actions of insulin.

Metabolic actions
Suppression of hepatic glucose production
Stimulation of glucose uptake by muscle (and adipose tissue)
Promotion of glucose storage as glycogen
Suppression of adipocyte lipolysis
Inhibition of ketogenesis
Regulation of protein turnover
Effects on electrolyte balance

Other actions
Regulation of growth and development (e.g. *in utero*)
Regulation of gene expression

transport and gene expression. The main actions of insulin are presented in Table 1.1. These include:
- Acute metabolic actions.
- Longer-term effects on growth and development.

Regulation of insulin secretion

Insulin is synthesized and secreted by the β-cells of the pancreatic islets in response to glucose and other secretagogues, such as amino acids. The secretion of insulin is very tightly matched to circulating glucose concentrations. Insulin is secreted at a low background (or basal) level throughout the day; this accounts for approximately 50% of insulin secretion. The remainder is secreted in close temporal association to the rise in portal plasma glucose following meals. Insulin secretion is inhibited by some other hormones, notably adrenaline (epinephrine) and somatostatin. By contrast, insulin secretion is enhanced by some other hormones (e.g. glucagon). Insulin may also exert autocrine effects, inhibiting its own secretion.

Counter-regulatory hormones

The metabolic actions of insulin are antagonized by the so-called counter-regulatory hormones:

* Glucagon.
* Catecholamines.
* Cortisol.
* Growth hormone.

These hormones enter their anti-insulin actions through direct tissue effects and, in the case of the catecholamines, indirectly by inhibition of insulin secretion.

Insulin biosynthesis

The preproinsulin gene is located on the short arm of chromosome 11. Transcription produces the precursor preproinsulin which is cleaved by a peptidase to proinsulin. Within the Golgi, proinsulin is converted via intermediates to the final secretory products insulin and C (connecting) peptide (Fig. 1.2). Insulin and C peptide are released in equimolar quantities when insulin secretory granules fuse with the cell membrane, releasing their contents. Within the β-cell insulin, molecules associate as hexameric crystals around two zinc ions.

1.2.2 The insulin receptor

Structure of the insulin receptor

The actions of insulin are mediated via binding of the hormone to receptors located in the membrane of almost all

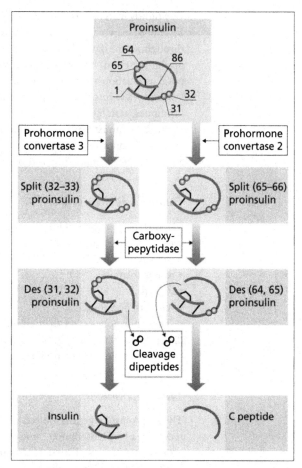

Fig. 1.2 Steps in insulin biosynthesis and processing. C-peptide is released in equimolar amounts with insulin. The plasma concentrations of less active precursors (proinsulin and split proinsulin molecules) is normally < 10% than that of insulin. (Redrawn with permission from S. Howell. In: Pickup, J.C. & Williams, G. 1997. *Textbook of Diabetes*, 2nd edn, Blackwell Science, Oxford.)

mammalian cells (Fig. 1.3); the receptor binds insulin with high affinity and specificity. The insulin receptor consists of two 135 kDa α-subunits and two 95 kDa β-subunits covalently linked by disulphide bonds to form a tetrameric glycoprotein complex (β–α–α–β). The insulin receptor gene is located on the short arm of chromosome 19, close

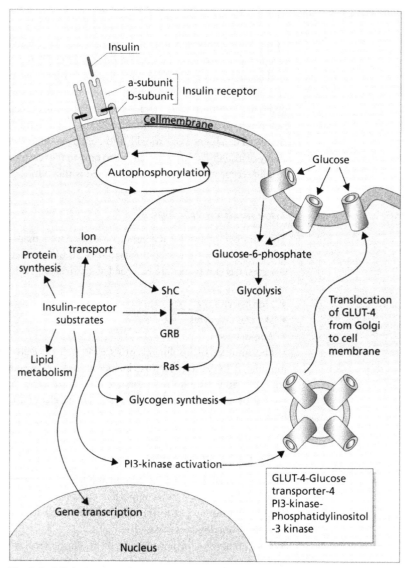

Fig. 1.3 Cellular binding of insulin to its receptor and key post-binding events. Following insulin binding, the β-subunit of the insulin receptor is autophosphorylated on tyrosine residues. Insulin receptor substrates (IRS-1–4) are the primary targets for phosphorylation by the activated receptor. In turn this permits propagation of the insulin signal via interactions with other proteins. Insulin-stimulated glucose entry into cells is facilitated by GLUT-4 glucose transporters, via activation of PI3-kinase. Phosphorylation of Shc leads to formation of an Shc-GRB-2 complex which activates the ras pathway; this results ultimately in glycogen synthesis via dephosphorylation and activation of glycogen synthase. (Redrawn with permission from Krentz, A.J. 2000. *Churchill's Pocketbook of Diabetes*. Churchill Livingstone, Edinburgh.)

to the low-density lipoprotein receptor gene. The insulin receptor gene spans > 150 kb, comprising 22 exons separated by long introns. Differential splicing of exon 11 yields two distinct mRNA species which encode α-subunits with different C-terminal tails. Tissue-specific expression of these isoforms have been identified which differ in insulin-binding affinity. The absence of exon 11 also confers an increased ability of insulin-like growth factor-1 to bind to the receptor. Insulin receptor biosynthesis is completed within 3 h.

Tissue insulin receptor expression

The number of insulin receptors varies between tissues, being as low as < 50 per erythrocyte to > 20 000 on hepatocytes. Certain tissues are regarded as classical targets for insulin:
- Hepatocytes.
- Skeletal myocytes.
- Adipocytes.

The number of insulin receptors expressed on cells is modulated by various factors, including ambient insulin concentrations. Insulin receptors are internalized and degraded by endocytosis; these processes are accelerated by insulin.

1.2.3 Post-binding events

Binding of insulin to the α-subunit induces a conformational change which has two important effects:
- The inhibitory effect of the α-subunit on the β-subunit autophosphorylation is released.
- The affinity for further binding of insulin molecules is reduced.

Autophosphorylation at multiple tyrosine sites within the transmembrane β-subunit of the receptor is a key element in insulin signalling (Fig. 1.3). In turn, this leads to a cascade of post-receptor signalling events which remain only partially elucidated. Insulin-receptor substrate-1, which together with insulin-receptor substrate-2 is expressed in skeletal muscle, is phosphorylated on tyrosine residues by the activated insulin receptor. The insulin-receptor substrates function as docking proteins to which many diverse proteins bind non-covalently through specific (src homo-logy 2) domains. The latter include phosphatidylinositol 3-kinase (essential for insulin-stimulated glucose transport; see below). Subsequent phosphorylation/dephosphorylation cascades lead ultimately to the activation of key enzymes, such as glycogen synthase and pyruvate dehydrogenase. Impaired actions of insulin may result from two main mechanisms.

1 *Receptor defects:* a reduced number of insulin receptors or a reduction in their affinity for insulin. This may occur in response to chronic hyperinsulinaemia (so-called down-regulation). Lesser degrees of obesity and glucose intolerance (see Section 2.5.4) are associated with receptor defects which may be largely reversible with treatment. Inherited severe receptor defects are rare (see Section 2.4).

2 *Post-binding defects:* defects in intracellular events distal to the binding of insulin account for insulin resistance in most patients with type 2 diabetes. The maximal response to insulin is impaired and is usually only partially reversible, even with the insulin-sensitizing thiazolidinediones (see Section 3). The precise nature of these defects has not yet been identified.

1.2.4 Glucose metabolism

In healthy individuals, plasma glucose concentrations are strictly maintained in the range of approximately 4–7 mmol/L (70–125 mg/dL). At any time point, the plasma glucose concentration reflects the net balance between:
• Rate of appearance of glucose in the circulation.
• Rate of disappearance from the circulation.

The glucose-lowering effects of insulin (Fig. 1.4) result primarily from two actions.

1 *Suppression of endogenous glucose production* (i.e. reducing the rate of glucose release into the blood).

2 *Stimulation of glucose disposal,* principally by skeletal muscle and, to a lesser degree, adipose tissue (i.e. increasing clearance from the circulation).

Endogenous glucose production

In the post-absorptive state (i.e. after an overnight fast) the

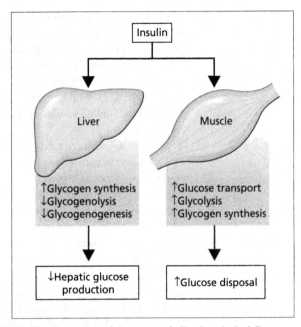

Fig. 1.4 Regulation of glucose metabolism by principal direct effects of insulin. (Redrawn with permission from Krentz, A.J. 2000. *Churchill's Pocketbook of Diabetes.* Churchill Livingstone, Edinburgh.)

Hepatic glucose production is the principal determinant of fasting blood glucose concentration

rate at which glucose enters the circulation from the liver is the main determinant of plasma glucose concentrations. This glucose is derived from breakdown of stored glycogen and synthesis of *de novo* glucose molecules from 3-carbon precursors (gluconeogenesis). As glycogen stores become depleted, gluconeogenesis assumes a quantitatively greater role. Suppression of hepatic glucose production is a major regulatory action of insulin. Glucagon is the main hormone accelerating hepatic glucose production. Renal gluconeogenesis also contributes to endogenous glucose production, accounting for approximately 25% of the total.

Glucose disposal

Stimulation of glucose uptake (and subsequent metabolism or storage as glycogen) requires higher plasma insulin

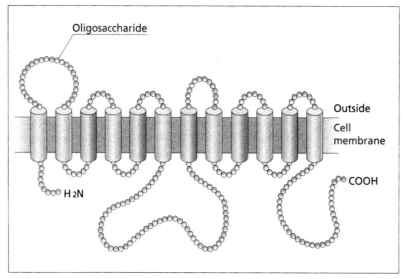

Fig. 1.5 Predicted structure of a glucose transporter protein. (Redrawn with permission from Kruzynska, Y. 1997. In: Pickup, J.C. & Williams, G. *Textbook of Diabetes*, 2nd edn. Blackwell Science, Oxford.)

Table 1.2 The glucose transporter protein family.

	K_m	Tissue location	Characteristics
GLUT-1	20	Fetal tissues, brain, kidney	Constitutive glucose transporter
GLUT-2	40	Liver, kidney, β-cell	Low-affinity glucose transporter
GLUT-3	10	Neurones, placenta	High-affinity glucose transporter
GLUT-4	2–10	Skeletal muscle, heart muscle, adipose tissue	Insulin-responsive glucose transporter
GLUT-7	?	Hepatocytes	Endoplasmic reticulum

K_m, Michaelis–Menten constant; GLUT-5 is a fructose transporter.

concentrations than are necessary for suppression of hepatic glucose production. A major action of insulin is to stimulate translocation of facilitative glucose transporters (GLUT-4) from intracellular pools to the cell membrane (Fig. 1.5). Other isoforms of glucose transporters (e.g. GLUT-1 at the blood–brain and blood–retinal barriers, GLUT-2 in islet β-cells) do not require insulin to transfer glucose into cells (Table 1.2). In the basal state, i.e. after an overnight fast, the majority of glucose (approximately 80%) is utilized via insulin-independent pathways by tissues with obligatory glucose requirements. These include the central and peripheral nervous systems, erythrocytes, leucocytes and renal medulla (Fig. 1.5).

Defects in GLUT-4 function are thought to be crucial to the insulin resistance that characterizes obesity, type 2 diabetes and the insulin resistance (metabolic) syndrome. Translocation of GLUT-4 can be stimulated by insulin or directly through non-insulin-dependent mechanisms including:

• Physical exercise.
• Insulin-like growth factor-1.
• Thyroid hormones.

Indirect pathways may also result in enhanced GLUT-4 translocation, including sulphonylurea therapy (see Section 3.2.3) and possibly leptin (see Section 1.6.2).

The Cori cycle

Lactate and hydrogen ions (H^+) are the products of anaerobic glycolysis, the reaction of which can be summarized as:

$$glucose \rightarrow 2 \, lactate^- + 2 \, H^+.$$

The principal lactic acid-producing organs are:
• Skeletal muscle.
• Brain.
• Erythrocytes.
• Renal medulla.

The liver, kidneys and heart normally extract lactate but may become net producers of lactic acid under conditions of severe ischaemia. Lactate produced by glycolysis may be completely oxidized to CO_2 and water in the tricarboxylic acid cycle, thereby consuming an equimolar amount of hydrogen ions:

$$lactate^- + 3 \, O_2 + H^+ \rightarrow 3 \, CO_2 + 3 \, H_2O.$$

Alternatively, lactate may enter the gluconeogenesis pathway in the liver and kidney to reform glucose; this step completes the Cori cycle:

$$2 \, lactate^- + 2 \, H^+ \rightarrow glucose.$$

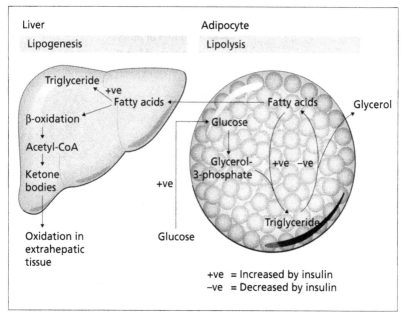

Fig. 1.6 Regulation of lipolysis and ketone body metabolism by insulin. (Adapted with permission from Krentz, A.J. 2000. *Churchill's Pocketbook of Diabetes*. Churchill Livingstone, Edinburgh.)

1.2.5 Lipid metabolism

Insulin plays a crucial role in inhibiting the hydrolysis of adipose tissue stores of triglyceride to non-esterified fatty acids (plus the gluconeogenic precursor, glycerol). In addition to reducing lipolysis via effects on the enzyme hormone-sensitive lipase (Fig. 1.6), insulin promotes glucose uptake by adipocytes, thereby promoting re-esterification via increased availability of glycerol-3-phosphate. Inhibition of lipolysis occurs at low-physiological insulin concentrations. Thus, increments of 60–90 pmol/L (10–15 mU/L) above fasting plasma insulin levels are normally sufficient to prevent hydrolysis of triglycerides (Fig. 1.7).

Adipocyte lipolysis is normally very sensitive to suppression by insulin

Fatty acids are the principal substrate for ketogenesis within the liver. Within the hepatocyte, the balance between insulin and glucagon concentrations regulates the fate of fatty acids. A high insulin : glucagon ratio favours re-esterification; a low ratio (typically found in patients with diabetic ketoacidosis) diverts fatty acids into the

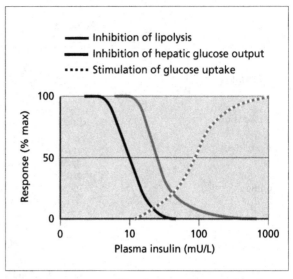

Fig. 1.7 Dose–response effects for the major metabolic actions of insulin. Note that for endogenous insulin portal blood concentrations are approximately twofold higher reflecting hepatic clearance of insulin. (Redrawn with permission from Kruzynska, Y. 1997. In: Pickup, J.C. & Williams, G. *Textbook of Diabetes*, 2nd edn. Blackwell Science, Oxford.)

Insulin has anti-ketogenic actions

intramitochondrial β-oxidation pathway leading to ketone body formation. Thus, via control of plasma fatty acid levels and other effects, insulin is a major regulator of ketogenesis (Fig. 1.6). Both fatty acids and ketones can be used as alternative fuels, e.g. during starvation and prolonged exercise. Insulin also increases the disposal of ketone bodies in extra-hepatic tissues.

1.2.6 Protein metabolism

Insulin regulates protein metabolism, stimulating tissue uptake of insulin-sensitive amino acids and transcription and translation of cellular proteins. Insulin also inhibits the breakdown of structural proteins.

Insulin has anabolic effects on protein metabolism

The tissue wasting characteristic of uncontrolled type 1 diabetes testifies to the importance of the anabolic effects of insulin on protein metabolism. Quantitatively, alanine is the most important gluconeogenic amino acid.

1.2.7 Ion transport

Hyperinsulinaemia acutely stimulates renal sodium retention. This mechanism has been invoked in insulin resistance-associated hypertension (see Section 2.5.7), although its relevance remains uncertain.

Potassium transport into cells is stimulated by insulin, the maximal effect occurring at pharmacological plasma insulin concentrations.

Insulin regulates sodium and potassium transport

1.3 The concept of insulin resistance

Reduced sensitivity of target tissues to the actions of insulin (effectively the reciprocal of insulin resistance) was originally postulated over 60 years ago before the advent of insulin immunoassays.

1.3.1 Early studies of insulin action

The pioneering studies of Himsworth at London University during the 1930s laid the foundations for our present views of insulin action. In a series of studies, Himsworth introduced the first standardized approach to quantifying insulin sensitivity *in vivo*. Two oral glucose tolerance tests, one with and one without a dose of exogenous insulin, were performed in diabetic subjects. Examination of the plasma glucose responses allowed the identification of two subtypes: insulin-sensitive and insulin-insensitive, the latter predominating. The clinical characteristics of the insulin-insensitive subjects suggest that they would be classified today as having type 2 diabetes. A deficiency of an unidentified insulin-sensitizing factor was postulated. Incidentally, Himsworth argued against use of the term 'insulin resistance'. The concept of decreased sensitivity to exogenous insulin was to be expanded and refined by later investigators. This required the development of methods allowing the measurement of insulin concentrations in plasma.

1.3.2 Radioimmunoassays for insulin

More direct evidence of insulin insensitivity was obtained in the 1960s following the development of a

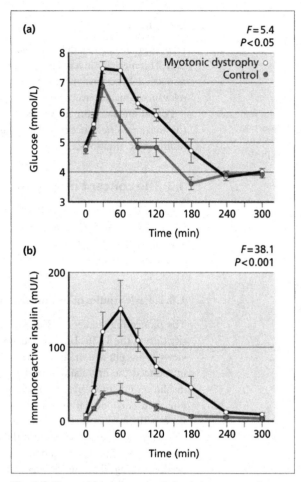

Fig. 1.8 Venous blood glucose and plasma immunoreactive insulin responses to a 75-g oral glucose tolerance test in patients with myotonic dystrophy and healthy control subjects matched for age, sex and body mass index. *F*-values indicate overall differences between the groups by two-way analysis of variance. (Redrawn with permission from Krentz, A.J. *et al.* 1990. *Metabolism* **39**, 938–942.) To convert to pmol/L, multiply by 6. To convert to mg/dL, multiply by 18.

radioimmunoassay for insulin. Yalow and Berson demonstrated an exaggerated and delayed response to an oral glucose challenge in diabetic subjects. As concomitant hyperglycaemia was observed it was concluded that these subjects were relatively insensitive to insulin. Similar observations have been made in many subsequent studies involving different groups of insulin-resistant subjects with or without diabetes (Fig. 1.8). Yalow and Berson also reported a hyperinsulinaemic response in obese non-diabetic subjects. However, the oral glucose tolerance test is an imperfect and indirect method for assessing the degree of insulin resistance.

Limitations of conventional radioimmunoassays have led to refinements in insulin assays (see section 1.5.1).

1.4 Definitions of insulin resistance

Building on Himsworth's original concept, Berson and Yalow later defined insulin resistance as:

> 'A state in which greater than normal amounts of insulin are required to elicit a quantitatively normal response.'

This definition presupposes that a normal response can ultimately be attained if sufficient insulin is present. The introduction of more sophisticated techniques for the assessment of insulin action led to Ronald Kahn's (1978) proposal that insulin resistance could be regarded in a more generic sense, existing whenever:

> 'Normal concentrations of insulin produce a less than normal biological response.'

This definition has two particular attractions:

• It implies the importance of performing studies at physiologically relevant insulin concentrations.
• It does not restrict consideration of insulin resistance to a single facet of metabolism.

Thus, impaired insulin action can be considered in relation to glucose and lipid metabolism, ion transport, protein synthesis, endothelial function, gene transcription, etc. (Table 1.1). However, the main focus of interest has remained the effects of insulin as the principal hormonal regulator of glucose metabolism.

Insulin sensitivity and insulin responsiveness

Kahn went on to subdivide insulin resistance into two components, based on observations that maximal effects of insulin on glucose metabolism requires occupation

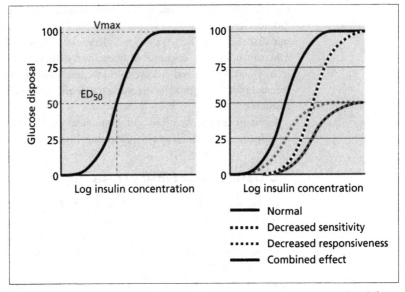

Fig. 1.9 Insulin resistance—theoretical effects of insulin receptor and post-binding defects. The receptor defect shows a rightward displacement from the normal sigmoidal dose–response curve. However, a 100% maximal response is still obtained. By contrast, a post-receptor defect limits the maximal effect that can be attained. Combined defects result in further impairment of insulin action. (Redrawn with permission from Kahn, C.R. 1978. *Metabolism* **27** (suppl 2), 1893–1902.)

of only a fraction of available cellular insulin receptors (Fig. 1.9).

• *Insulin responsiveness:* the maximal effect that can be achieved (V_{max} according to Michaelis–Menten kinetics).

• *Insulin sensitivity:* the dose–response that exists between an absence of effect and the maximal effect quantified as the concentration of insulin which produces a half-maximal response (ED_{50}).

Kahn argued that reduced sensitivity—i.e. a right-shift in the dose–response curve—would result from defects at the level of the interaction of insulin with its specific receptor (Fig. 1.9). Conversely, decreased responsiveness would reflect a rate-limiting defect(s) beyond the receptor, i.e. post-receptor (or post-binding). Mixed defects could also occur. This framework has provided insights into defective insulin action in obesity, glucose intolerance and type 2 diabetes (see Section 2).

1.5 Assessment of insulin action *in vivo*

Metabolic investigations are usually performed in the post-absorptive state, i.e. after an overnight fast (8–12h). To minimize acute metabolic perturbations preparation of subject should include:
• Abstinence from alcohol and tobacco for the preceding 24 h.
• Minimal physical exercise (including the morning of the study—subjects should not cycle and should arrive by transport).
• Avoidance of caffeine on morning of study—caffeine causes release of catecholamines and may acutely impair insulin action.
• Minimization of discomfort—consider use local anaesthetic for intravenous cannulation. Avoid excessive noise and distraction during studies.
• Avoidance of mental stress during study.e.g. puzzle solving, mental arithmetic.

Health control subjects should have no impairment of liver or kidney function, no history of hypertension or dyslipidaemia and should not be taking drugs with metabolic actions. Avoid studies for 6–8 weeks following acute servere illness or surgery.

1.5.1 Fasting insulin concentration

If islet β-cell function is unimpaired, insulin resistance in target tissues is normally compensated for by increased endogenous insulin secretion. Thus, normoglycaemia (or hyperglycaemia) in the presence of hyperinsulinaemia provides prima-facie evidence of insulin resistance; Fig. 1.10 illustrates this principle.

Measurement of fasting plasma glucose and insulin concentrations following an overnight fast minimizes the confounding effect of changes in blood glucose that occur after meals. Although this approach provides at best only an estimate of insulin sensitivity the simplicity of sampling lends itself to epidemiological studies. Interpretation of fasting hyperinsulinaemia is hampered by the following limitations.
• Overlap between normal and elevated insulin concentrations between insulin-sensitive and insulin-resistant

Normoglycaemia or hyperglycaemia with hyperinsulinaemia denotes insulin resistance

19

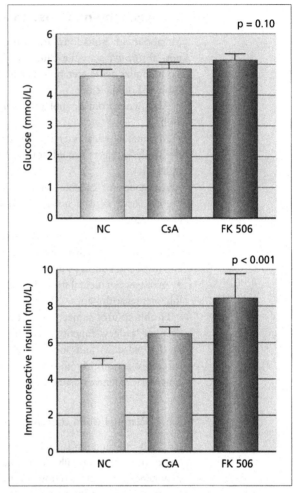

Fig. 1.10 Fasting blood glucose and plasma immunoreactive insulin concentrations (mean ± SE) in three groups of subjects ($n = 10$ for each). The CsA and FK506 groups were liver transplant recipients randomized to immunosuppressive treatment with cyclosporin A and FK506 (tacrolimus), respectively. NC = normal controls. The three groups were matched for age, sex and body mass index. The *P*-values denote differences between the three groups by one-way analysis of variance. Plasma immunoreactive insulin concentrations were significantly higher in the CsA- ($P < 0.01$) and FK506-treated patients ($P < 0.02$) than the controls. (Data with permission from Krentz, A.J. *et al.* 1993. *Diabetes* **42**, 1753–1759.) To convert to pmol/L, multiply by 6. To convert to mg/dL, multiply by 18.

individuals. This extends to more direct measures of insulin resistance (see Section 2.2.1). Reaven has shown that some otherwise healthy individuals have degrees of insulin resistance similar to those typical of patients with glucose intolerance or type 2 diabetes.

• Cross-reactivity of proinsulin and partially processed proinsulin molecules in many standard radioimmunoassays. The proportion of these molecules secreted in relation to insulin is increased in some states of insulin resistance, including impaired glucose tolerance and type 2 diabetes (see Fig. 1.2). Proinsulin-like molecules have approximately 10% of the activity of insulin. Thus the true level of hyperinsulinaemia may be somewhat overestimated unless more specific two-site immunoradiometric assays are employed (Fig. 1.11).

• Absence of a standardized insulin assay permitting reliable comparisons between laboratories.

Assumptions about insulin clearance are integral to this approach. Measurement of plasma C-peptide—which is secreted on an equimolar basis with insulin but is not subject to hepatic clearance—is an attractive alternative (Fig. 1.11). However, there is much less data available on C-peptide as a marker of endogenous insulin secretion.

Clinical significance of hyperinsulinaemia

Hyperinsulinaemia has been identified in epidemiological studies as a risk marker for:

• *Type 2 diabetes*. Elevated plasma insulin concentrations, whether fasting or following a glucose challenge, are a powerful predictor of type 2 diabetes, independently of obesity. The risk is particularly marked for individuals with a first-degree relative with diabetes.

• *Cardiovascular disease*. Hyperinsulinaemia has also been identified as a risk marker for atherosclerotic disease in several prospective studies. However, the nature and strength of the association has been inconsistent between studies. Because of these caveats, measurement of fasting plasma insulin concentration is not currently recommended in the assessment of cardiovascular risk in clinical practice.

Some of the most convincing evidence comes from the Quebec study in 2103 non-diabetic men (Fig. 1.12) which

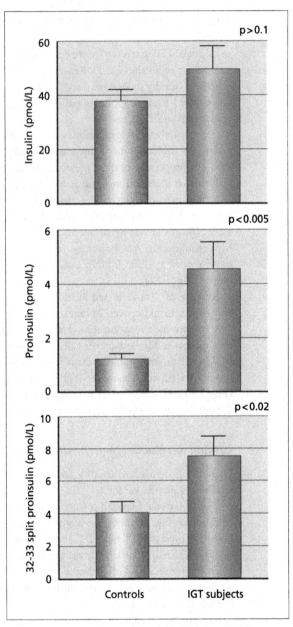

Fig. 1.11 Fasting plasma insulin, proinsulin and 32–33 split proinsulin concentrations (mean ± SE) in non-obese men with recently diagnosed impaired glucose tolerance (IGT) and healthy controls ($n = 8$ for each) matched for age and body mass index. Plasma immunoreactive insulin concentrations were significantly higher in the subjects with IGT (7.4 ± 1.0 vs. 2.9 ± 0.3, $P < 0.05$) whereas C-peptide concentrations were similar (0.70 ± 0.09 vs. 0.52 ± 0.05, $P > 0.1$). The two-site immunoradiometric assays indicate that the degree of hyperinsulinaemia was overestimated by cross-reactivity between proinsulin-like molecules in the immunoassay. (Data with permission from Krentz, A.J. *et al.* 1991. *Diabetic Medicine* **8**, 848–854 and Krentz, A.J. *et al.* 1993. *Clinical Science* **85**, 97–100.) To convert to mU/L, divide by 6.0.

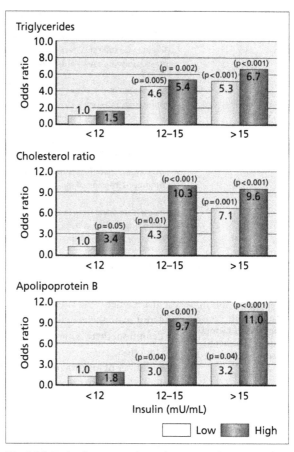

Fig. 1.12 Ratios for coronary heart disease according to baseline fasting insulin, triglycerides, total : HDL-cholesterol ratio and apolipoprotein B concentrations in non-diabetic men followed for 5 years. (Redrawn with permission from Després, J.-P. *et al*. 1996. *New England Journal of Medicine* **334**, 952–957.)

Hyperinsulinaemia has been identified as a marker for cardiovascular disease

employed an insulin assay with no significant cross-reactivity with proinsulin. This study also included detailed assessment of plasma lipids (a potential confounding influence not always accounted for in other studies). Concomitant elevation of apoprotein B in men with the greatest hyperinsulinaemia increased the risk of coronary heart disease synergistically (Fig. 1.12).

As β-cell dysfunction frequently coexists with impaired insulin action, more rigorous evaluation of insulin action is

Table 1.3 Techniques for the assessment of insulin action *in vivo*.

Dynamic techniques—endogenous insulin
Oral glucose tolerance test
Intravenous glucose tolerance test
Dynamic techniques—exogenous insulin
Insulin tolerance test
Incremental insulin infusion
Mathematical modelling techniques
Minimal model (of Bergman)
Homeostasis model assessment
Continuous infusion of glucose with model assessment
Steady-state open-loop techniques
Insulin suppression test
Euglycaemic hyperinsulinaemic glucose clamp

Hyperglycaemia in concert with hyperinsulinaemia implies a defect in insulin secretion

required, particularly if there is any degree of hyperglycaemia. Under these circumstances, hyperinsulinaemia will underestimate the magnitude of insulin resistance because, by definition, there is inevitably also some impairment of β-cell function.

A number of investigative techniques have been devised, each of which has particular limitations; none is suitable for routine clinical use (Table 1.3).

1.5.2 Dynamic techniques—endogenous insulin

In these techniques, glucose metabolism is perturbed, by design, through stimulation of endogenous insulin secretion.

Oral glucose tolerance test

This is subject to some of the limitations of the aforementioned closed-loop feedback that exists between the islet β-cell and target tissues. The higher the glucose : insulin ratio, the greater the degree of insulin resistance. Other drawbacks include:
- The potential influence of variable rates of gastric emptying.
- The incretin effect of gastrointestinal glucose delivery (which results in greater insulin response than intravenous glucose). See also section 1.5.4.

Intravenous glucose tolerance test

This is discussed in Section 1.5.3 (the minimal model of Bergman). This technique is also used to assess insulin secretion.

1.5.3 Dynamic techniques—exogenous insulin

Insulin tolerance test

In the insulin tolerance test, which risks inducing unpleasant hypoglycaemia, the fall in blood glucose to an intravenous bolus of insulin reflects the net effects on the liver and peripheral tissues. Plasma glucose concentration is measured every 5 min allowing a log–linear decline to be plotted, the slope of which (k_{ITT}) may be calculated. However:

• Localization of defective insulin action, i.e. liver vs. muscle, is not possible using this approach.

• Glucagon, catecholamines, cortisol and growth hormone, secreted in response to hypoglycaemia, antagonize the actions of insulin at cellular level. Catecholamines also inhibit endogenous insulin secretion.

A shortened version of the technique has been developed which avoids both the unphysiological peak of insulin following injection and the confounding effects of counterregulatory hormone response to hypoglycaemia.

Low-dose incremental insulin infusion

In this technique, insulin is infused intravenously in hourly increments at doses of 0 (basal), 0.005, 0.01 and 0.05 U/kg/h. Blood glucose, fatty acids and other insulin-sensitive metabolites are permitted to decline in response to the graded hyperinsulinaemia. Blood samples are withdrawn at 10 min intervals during the final 30 min of each period. Dose–response relationships between insulin and the metabolite of interest are examined and the displacement between mean regression lines is examined using statistical methods (Fig. 1.13). The technique can be combined with isotopic glucose turnover using the non-steady state equations of Steele *et al*. As plasma insulin concentra-

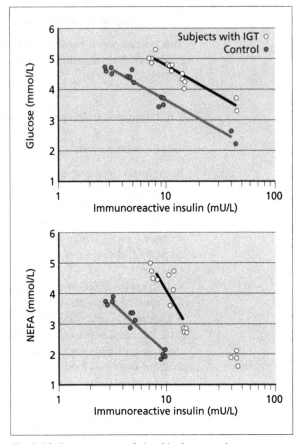

Fig. 1.13 Dose–response relationships between plasma immunoreactive insulin vs. blood glucose and plasma non-esterified fatty acids in non-obese men ($n = 8$) with impaired glucose tolerance and matched healthy controls derived from low-dose incremental insulin infusions. Data points represent group mean values at each sampling time point. Significant rightward displacements ($P < 0.001$) were observed for each metabolite for the subjects with impaired glucose tolerance. (Redrawn with permission from Krentz, A.J. 1991. *Diabetic Medicine* **8**, 848–854.)

tions are confined to the low-physiological range the incremental infusion technique is appropriate for assessing lipolysis in insulin-resistant states. The decline in blood glucose primarily reflects suppression of hepatic glucose production rather than stimulation of glucose uptake. Limitations include:

• Hypoglycaemia may be induced in normal subjects during the highest infusion rate (see above, intravenous gluose tolerance test). This can be avoided by curtailing the study at the end of the 0.01 U/kg h infusion.

1.5.4 Mathematical modelling techniques

These techniques also utilize the closed-loop relationship between insulin secretion and insulin action.

Homeostasis model assessment

The Oxford group have applied mathematical modelling to basal concentrations of glucose and insulin (homeostasis model assessment). This approach provides an index of relative insulin sensitivity (R). The latter is derived from a single pair of values for each variable. The method is straightforward technically but has the following disadvantages.
• As insulin levels are confined to fasting levels, insulin-stimulated glucose disposal, which occurs at higher insulin concentrations (Fig. 1.7), cannot be reliably assessed.
• The technique is highly dependent on the assumptions of the model and precision of the insulin assay.

Continuous infusion of glucose with model assessment

Similar limitations apply to the technique of continuous infusion of glucose with model assessment. Endogenous insulin secretion is stimulated using a 60-min infusion of glucose (5 mg/kg/min). Comparability with the glucose clamp technique (see Section 1.5.6) has been reported; however:
• The site of insulin resistance (hepatic vs. muscle) cannot be identified.
• The between-day coefficient of variation is reported to be approximately 20%.

The minimal model (of Bergman)

The frequently sampled intravenous glucose tolerance test utilizes a rapid intravenous injection of glucose from which the glucose disappearance curve may be derived using two differential equations as devised by Bergman *et al.* The so-

The minimal model uses a simplified representation of glucose kinetics to provide an insulin sensitivity index

called minimal model is based on assumptions about glucose distribution and the mechanisms of glucose disposal.

One equation represents glucose kinetics (assuming a single compartment model for glucose distribution) whereas the other describes the effects of insulin (which is assumed to occur in a remote compartment). The model predicts plasma glucose concentrations at various time points from the measured insulin levels according to preset parameters of glucose metabolism and kinetics and action of insulin. The predicted values are compared with the measured plasma glucose concentrations and the parameters are altered until the error between estimated and measured plasma glucose values is minimized. In non-diabetic subjects, the index of insulin sensitivity (S_I) reportedly correlates well with the M-value (reflecting insulin-mediated glucose disposal) derived from the glucose clamp technique. The minimal model also permits an assessment of the ability of glucose to promote its own clearance independently of insulin; this is known as glucose effectiveness (S_G). However:

• Because the intravenous glucose tolerance test relies on adequate endogenous insulin secretion, the coadministration of a sulphonylurea (tolbutamide) is sometimes necessary in patients with type 2 diabetes.

• It has been argued that S_G must reflect basal insulin-mediated glucose clearance (see Section 1.2.4) in addition to insulin-independent glucose uptake.

Although certain biases are inherent, which place some limitations on the validity of the minimal model, the relative simplicity of the technique has helped to ensure its widespread application.

Oral glucose tolerance test

Mari *et al.* have described a model based on the 75 g oral glucose tolerance test. Preliminary studies suggest reasonable correlations with other techniques. Further evaluation is required.

1.5.5 Insulin suppression test

Pharmacological interruption of the aforementioned physiological feedback loop allows insulin-stimulated glucose disposal to be isolated and quantified under steady-state conditions. In the original quadruple infusion version, devised by Reaven *et al.* at Stanford University, the insulin suppression test involved suppression of endogenous insulin secretion using adrenaline (epinephrine). A non-selective β-adrenergic blocker (propranolol) was coinfused to counter other metabolic effects of the adrenaline. However:

• Complete β-blockade could not be guaranteed.
• Cardiac dysrhythmias presented a potential hazard and so this approach was abandoned.

Later modifications of the technique used a constant infusion of somatostatin to suppress insulin (and glucagon) secretion. The other infusions are glucose and exogenous insulin which are infused at constant rates, producing plasma insulin concentrations of approximately 100 mU/L. Under these circumstances it is assumed that hepatic glucose production will be completely inhibited. Thus, the resulting mean steady-state plasma glucose concentration will reflect the sensitivity of extra-hepatic tissues to insulin; the higher the plasma glucose, the lower the insulin sensitivity. This technique provides data similar to that obtained using the glucose clamp at similar plasma insulin concentrations. Glucose clearance may be calculated by dividing the exogenous infusion rate by the steady-state plasma glucose concentration.

• Glycosuria may occur if the renal threshold for glucose is exceeded; renal losses must be subtracted from the glucose infusion rate.

1.5.6 Hyperinsulinaemic euglycaemic clamp technique

The hyperinsulinaemic euglycaemic clamp, which involves simultaneous intravenous infusions of insulin and hypertonic glucose, is widely regarded as the reference method for determining insulin action. Developed originally by Andres *et al.*, the technique has been extensively employed in human studies.

Briefly, if endogenous hepatic glucose production is completely inhibited by a continuous intravenous infusion of insulin ($40 \ mU/m^2/min$ or higher) then the quantity of

The glucose clamp technique is widely regarded as the reference method for assessing whole-body insulin action

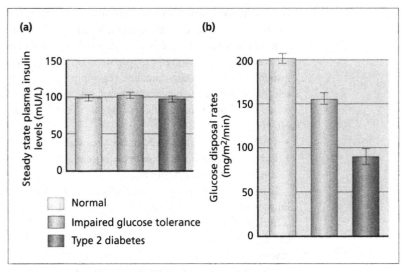

Fig. 1.14 (a) Mean (± SE) plasma immunoreactive insulin concentrations and (b) tissue glucose uptake for subjects with normal glucose tolerance and patients with impaired glucose tolerance and type 2 diabetes, respectively, as determined during euglycaemic hyperinsulinaemic clamps. Despite similar steady-state hyperinsulinaemia, glucose disposal rates were decreased by 24% in patients with impaired glucose tolerance and by 58% in the patients with type 2 diabetes. (Redrawn with permission from Kolterman, O.G. 1981. *Journal of Clinical Investigation* **68**, 957–969.) To convert to pmol/L, multiply by 6.

exogenous glucose required to maintain euglycaemia (the *M*-value) is a reflection of the net sensitivity of target tissues (mainly skeletal muscle; Fig. 1.3) to insulin. The *M*-value is determined when near steady-state has been attained; this requires several hours. In order to suppress hepatic glucose production, plasma insulin concentrations are typically raised from basal to approximately 600 pmol/L (100 mU/L) (Fig. 1.14). This is achieved by a primed-continuous infusion of soluble insulin. Plasma glucose is measured every 5 min and hypoglycaemia is avoided by concomitant infusion of variable rate hypertonic glucose. Usually, euglycaemia is the aim but the basic technique can also be used to 'clamp' the plasma glucose concentration at any desired level. Euglycaemia avoids confounding effects of either hypoglycaemia (causing counter-regulatory hormone secretion) or hyperglycaemia (which may result in urinary glucose losses).

Multiple studies, carried out on separate days and conducted at different plasma insulin concentrations, allow construction of whole-body dose–response curves analogous to the Kahn model (see Fig. 1.9). This permits evaluation of binding vs. post-binding defects. However, the glucose clamp technique has tended to diminish the concept of insulin resistance to a reduced M-value. Indeed, a reduced rate of insulin-mediated glucose disposal has come to be regarded as virtually synonymous with insulin resistance. The limitations of the clamp technique require acknowledgement:

- Not only is the sustained hyperinsulinaemia attained in most clamp studies unphysiological but it is also inappropriate for the assessment of other key aspects of intermediary metabolism. Examination of Fig. 1.7 demonstrates that the glucose clamp technique is ideal for identifying impaired steady-state insulin-stimulated glucose disposal. However, because adipocyte lipolysis is regulated at plasma insulin levels in the low-physiological range (Fig. 1.7), this aspect of metabolism will be maximally suppressed in the early stages of a clamp. Performing glucose clamps at lower plasma insulin concentrations allows lipolysis to be assessed (Fig. 1.15).

- A similar caveat pertains to the assessment of hepatic glucose production, defects in the suppression of which will tend to be overlooked by standard clamp protocols. In fact, isotopic tracer studies suggest that suppression of hepatic glucose production is less effective in subjects with impaired glucose tolerance or type 2 diabetes, i.e. there is hepatic insulin resistance.

- Saturation of interstitial fluid with insulin may lead to higher rates of glucose disposal per increment in plasma insulin concentration.

- The technique is labour-intensive and operator-dependent.

The glucose clamp technique assesses whole-body insulin-mediated glucose disposal

1.5.7 Complementary techniques

The glucose clamp technique may be usefully combined with a number of complementary investigative techniques.

Insulin receptor binding studies

In vitro studies of the binding of insulin to purified receptors have provided additional insights into defective insulin

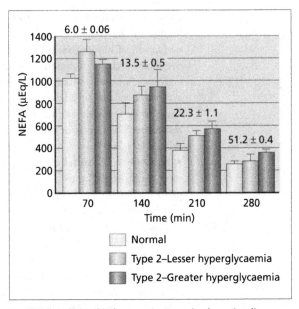

Fig. 1.15 Relationship between increases in plasma insulin concentration and non-esterified fatty acids during 70-min sequential infusion studies. The numbers above the bars represent the mean insulin concentration at the end of each infusion. Subjects are normal controls and patients with type 2 diabetes having either lesser (stippled bars) or greater degrees of hyperglycaemia. (Redrawn with permission from Swislocki, A.L.M. *et al.* 1987. *Diabetologia* **30**, 622–626.)

action in human disease. However, the physiological relevance of insulin receptor binding studies in non-classical target cells, such as erythrocytes, is questionable. A decrease in insulin receptor numbers has been reported in insulin-resistant states such as obesity (see Section 2.5.2) and impaired glucose tolerance (see Section 2.5.4). Defects of receptor autophosphorylation have been identified in patients with type 2 diabetes.

Indirect calorimetry

Indirect calorimetry comprises measurement of whole-body oxygen consumption and carbon dioxide generation to estimate:
• Energy metabolism.
• Substrate oxidation rates.

The technique can provide insights into the effects of insulin resistance on intracellular metabolism, e.g. the partition between glucose oxidation and glycogen synthesis in skeletal muscle. However, there are limitations inherent in the technique. First, the degree of hyperinsulinaemia generated in clamp studies may favour identification of defects in glucose storage rather than impaired glucose oxidation. Secondly, indirect calorimetry calculations rely on assumptions about the interrelationships between aspects of substrate utilization. Thus, while an inverse relationship exists between glucose and lipid oxidation it does not necessarily follow that oxidation of one substrate directly regulates the other. Finally, indirect calorimetry provides only an estimate of net changes in substrate oxidation.

Substrate balance studies

These were pioneered in the 1960s by Zierler and Rabinowitz who noted differences in insulin sensitivity between suppression of lipolysis and glucose uptake in the human forearm. By quantifying substrate utilization across a specific tissue bed, this relatively invasive technique provides more detailed information about the site of impaired insulin action, e.g. liver vs. skeletal muscle vs. adipose tissue. However, complete isolation of a particular organ or tissue is rarely possible and extrapolations to distant anatomical sites may have limited validity.

Biopsy techniques

These invasive techniques permit direct measurement of insulin-stimulated enzyme activity or mRNA levels in muscle or adipose tissue biopsies. Subcutaneous adipocytes are readily obtained under local anaesthetic from the lower abdominal wall. Visceral adipocytes may be obtained during surgical procedures. Vastus lateralis is the most commonly studied muscle (the potential for metabolic differences between anatomical sites must be considered). The samples can be used to study insulin binding, post-binding events, enzyme activities or glucose transporter function.

Adipose tissue microdialysis techniques

These are used to directly measure interstitial fluid concentrations of insulin and metabolites in subcutaneous adipose tissue and the responses to perturbations, such as a glucose clamp. It is noteworthy that in clamp studies the kinetics for changes in interstitial insulin concentrations are delayed by approximately 20 min compared with plasma levels.

Nuclear magnetic spectroscopy

This has been pioneered by Shulman *et al.* at Yale to measure insulin-stimulated glycogen synthesis in skeletal muscle. Intramuscular glucose and glucose-6-phosphate levels may be determined non-invasively, permitting identification of defects in glucose transport and metabolism.

Positron emission tomography

This imaging technique utilizes radiopharmaceuticals labelled with positron emitters. Appropriately labelled glucose, which is transported and phosphorylated but not metabolized further, has been used to investigate differences in substrate metabolism between skeletal and cardiac muscle. The scanners are presently available in only a few centres.

1.6 Mechanisms of insulin resistance

1.6.1 Genetic defects

It is widely accepted that insulin resistance often has a genetic component. In Pima Indians it has been estimated that approximately 30% of the variance in insulin sensitivity, as determined in glucose clamp studies, can be accounted for by familial clustering. However, many individual candidate gene loci for insulin resistance associated with type 2 diabetes have been excluded by linkage studies. These include those coding for insulin, glycogen synthase, GLUT-1, GLUT-4 and fatty-acid-binding protein 2. It is thought that a multiplicity of genes, the effects of which may be modulated by environmental factors, contribute to insulin resistance in its most commonly encountered forms, i.e. inheritance is polygenic. However, additional genetic or acquired defects of β-cell function are necessary for glucose intolerance to become manifest (see Section 2.5.5). Research has also been directed towards the regulatory sequences of candidate genes, e.g. studies of polymorphisms with variable-number tandem repeats near the insulin gene and its promoter. To date, studies in type 2 diabetes have been inconclusive, providing no clear evidence that this region is a major susceptibility locus. As insulin resistance and type 2 diabetes are closely associated with obesity, the recent identification of leptin and resistin (see Section 1.6.2) and the cloning of genes for uncoupling proteins are also attracting interest.

Insulin resistance is a complex genetic condition

Insulin receptor mutations

Rare mutations of the insulin receptor gene are the best characterized causes of intrinsic insulin resistance (see Section 2.4). Many different mutations have been described which may be classified functionally into the following classes.
- Class I—Decreased receptor biosynthesis
- Class II—Impaired post-translational processing
- Class III—Defects in insulin binding
- Class IV—Impaired tyrosine kinase activity

Impairment of insulin receptor intrinsic tyrosine kinase activity has been reported not only in subjects with type 2 diabetes but also in non-obese normoglycaemic individuals with insulin resistance. Type A extreme insulin resistance, some cases of which are caused by insulin receptor mutations, shares some metabolic and clinical features with the far more prevalent polycystic ovary syndrome (see Section 2.5.12).

Post-binding signalling mutations

Type C severe insulin resistance and many other uncommon or rare inherited insulin–resistance syndromes (see Section 2.4) result from post-binding defects in insulin signalling. In most, the precise sites of the defects remain undetermined. This is also the case for the common form of type 2 diabetes (see Section 2.5.5).

• *Insulin receptor substrate-1.* Mutations of the gene (mapped to chromosome 2q36) coding for insulin receptor substrate-1 have been sought in subjects with type 2 diabetes. A variant has been identified (a glycine–arginine substitution at codon 972), expression of which results in defective insulin signalling. However, the frequency of the variant has been found to be similar in patients with type 2 diabetes and non-diabetic controls.

• *Phosphatidylinositol-3 kinase.* Mutational analysis has shown that homozygous carriers of a mutation in the gene coding for phosphatidylinositol-3 kinase (affecting approximately 2% of white people) is impaired glucose tolerance and glucose effectiveness. The ~20% of white people who are heterozygous for the polymorphism are also relatively insulin resistant.

Genetic knockout animal models

'Knockout' mouse models with selective tissue deficiency of insulin receptors, insulin receptor substrate-1 or GLUT-4 have provided interesting insights into the aetiology of insulin resistance and type 2 diabetes. For example, selective deletion of islet β-cell insulin receptor substrate-1 causes loss of glucose sensing and progressive glucose intolerance. By contrast, mice deficient in GLUT-4 in all tissues show cardiac and adipose tissue abnormalities yet are not diabetic.

β_3-Adrenergic receptor mutations

The importance of mutations in the atypical β_3-adrenoceptor for defective insulin action in human is uncertain

In humans, β_3-adrenergic receptors are expressed mainly in visceral adipose tissue where they may contribute to the metabolic abnormalities associated with this form of obesity. In lower mammals the receptor is expressed in thermogenic brown adipose tissue. A mutation of the β_3-adrenergic receptor has been reported which is associated, albeit not strongly, with features of the insulin resistance syndrome and early onset of type 2 diabetes in Pima Indians. β_3-agonists have been developed as anti-obesity agents (see Section 3.3.4).

Calpain-10

Calpain-10, or cysteine protease, has been linked with type

2 diabetes in Mexican Americans. Identified by positional cloning the nature of the association is unclear and requires confirmation. Insulin resistance is a theoretical explanation for the association, but defective insulin secretion also appears possible.

1.6.2 Acquired forms of insulin resistance

Counter-regulatory hormones

Elevated levels of circulating hormones which antagonize the metabolic actions of insulin (see Section 1.2.1) are associated with impaired insulin action. These hormones, acting mainly at post-binding sites of insulin signalling, contribute to the acute insulin resistance associated with diabetic ketoacidosis, severe sepsis or major trauma (see Section 2.6.1). Specific hypersecretory endocrinopathies (see Section 2.6.2) are frequently associated with glucose intolerance or, less commonly, diabetes.

Drug therapy

Various drugs can influence insulin resistance: corticosteroids (dose-dependent effect); β-adrenergic blockers (especially agents without intrinsic β_2-agonist activity); and thiazide diuretics at higher doses. These are considered in more detail in Sections 2.7 and 3.5, respectively.

Glucose toxicity

Overactivity of the intracellular hexosamine pathway has been implicated in the detrimental effects of hyperglycaemia on:

• Endogenous insulin secretion.
• Glucose disposal.

These effects have been termed 'glucose toxicity'. The enzyme glutamine : fructose-6-phosphate amidotransferase diverts glucose away from glycolysis at the level of fructose-6-phosphate resulting in the formation of glucosamine-6-phosphate and other hexosamine products. The latter reduce GLUT-4 translocation in skeletal muscle. Transgenic mice overexpressing the enzyme are resistant to the

Reducing
hyperglycaemia
may lead to
secondary
improvements in
insulin secretion
and insulin action

actions of insulin on muscle glucose disposal. The clinical implication is that reducing the level of hyperglycaemia (whether by non-pharmacological measures, oral agents or insulin; see Section 3) may produce secondary improvements in insulin secretion and insulin action.

Glucose transporter defects

The role of defective insulin-sensitive glucose transporter protein (GLUT-4) function in type 2 diabetes has been clarified recently. The expression of GLUT-4 is reduced in adipocytes in subjects with obesity or type 2 diabetes. However, GLUT-4 expression is normal in skeletal muscle, the principal site for insulin-mediated glucose disposal. Defective translocation of GLUT-4 to the cell membrane has emerged as the most likely explanation for insulin resistance in muscle.

Lipotoxicity

Disturbed fatty acid metabolism has been documented in patients with type 2 diabetes and lesser degrees of glucose intolerance. Experimental data indicate that elevated fatty acid concentrations may:

- Impair insulin-mediated glucose disposal and oxidation.
- Accelerate hepatic glucose production.
- Inhibit endogenous insulin secretion.
- Contribute to hypertriglyceridaemia.

The glucose–fatty acid (or Randle) cycle was identified in isolated rat heart and diaphragm by Sir Philip Randle et al. in Cambridge, UK, in the early 1960s (Fig. 1.16). It was postulated that increased fat oxidation might cause the insulin resistance associated with diabetes and obesity.

Much evidence
supports the
existence of a
glucose–fatty acid
cycle

Increased fatty acids in muscle lead to a higher mitochondrial acetyl CoA : CoA ratio. This, in turn, inhibits pyruvate dehydrogenase activity with diversion of pyruvate to lactate or alanine rather than to acetyl CoA. Increased citrate levels inhibit phosphofructokinase activity leading to increased glucose-6-phosphate concentrations. Hexokinase is allosterically inhibited by the increased levels of glucose-6-phosphate and so reduced GLUT-4-mediated glucose

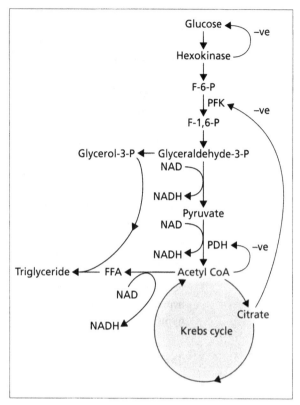

Fig. 1.16 The glucose–fatty acid (Randle) cycle. Potential enzymatic steps that might be influenced by free fatty acid (FFA) oxidation. NAD, nicotinamide adenine dinucleotide; PDH, pyruvate dehydrogenase; PFK, phosphofructokinase; G-6-P, glucose-6-phosphate; F-6-P, fructose-6-phosphate; F-1,6-P, fructose-1,6-bisphosphate. Modified with permission from Alzaid, A. & Rizza, R.A. (1993) In: *Insulin Resistance* (ed. D.E. Moller) John Wiley, Chichester.

transport/phosphorylation. Decreased glycogen synthase activity has also been reported. Thus:

- Skeletal glucose uptake is reduced.
- Glycolysis and glycogen synthesis is inhibited.

Recent observations in rats using magnetic resonance spectroscopy (see Section 1.5.7) suggest that reduced glucose transport is the main defect which leads to decreased glycogen synthesis and glucose oxidation. Fatty acid activation of protein kinase Cθ, a serine kinase, may also induce insulin resistance via reduced insulin receptor substrate-1.

Evidence for insulin resistance in the suppression of lipolysis with increased plasma fatty acid concentrations has attracted considerable attention. Reaven *et al.* have argued that failure of regulation of plasma fatty acid levels is a crucial determinant of hyperglycaemia in type 2 diabetes (see Section 2.5.5). Fatty acids normally stimulate glucose-mediated insulin secretion, thereby offsetting the adverse effects of elevated fatty acid concentrations on hepatic and peripheral glucose metabolism. However, if fatty acids fail to stimulate insulin secretion, hepatic glucose production will accelerate. This, in concert with a fatty-acid-induced reduction in glucose utilization, would result in hyperglycaemia. These effects may be regarded as evidence for a toxicity of fatty acids. Indeed, recent data suggest that under experimental conditions fatty acids may induce apoptosis (programmed cell death) in islet β-cells. In addition, elevated circulation fatty acid concentrations have also been implicated in the pathogenesis of some forms of hypertension via direct vascular effects and indirect mechanisms (see Section 2.5.7).

Fatty acids may induce apoptosis in islet β-cells

Tumour necrosis factor-α

The cytokine tumour necrosis factor-α, which is produced by adipocytes and immune cells, has been implicated in the production of insulin resistance via inhibitory effects on tyrosine kinase-mediated insulin signalling in skeletal muscle and adipose tissue (see section 2.5.2). Tumour necrosis factor-α signals through at least two known cell surface receptors. Expression of tumour necrosis-α, which exerts its effects through a paracrine mechanism, is high in obesity and type 2 diabetes. Circulating levels are low. Neutralization of tumour necrosis factor-α using monoclonal antibodies improves insulin resistance in the Zucker (*fa/fa*) rat. However, this effect has not been replicated in humans with type 2 diabetes.

Tumour necrosis factor-α levels are increased in obesity

Interleukins

Other cytokines, i.e. interleukins 1 and 6, in concert with other factors, control the centrally mediated stress response of severe sepsis or inflammation. The resulting activation of

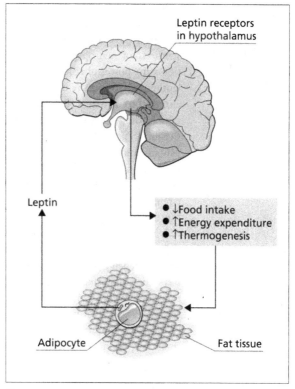

Leptin receptors
in hypothalamus

Leptin

• ↓Food intake
• ↑Energy expenditure
• ↑Thermogenesis

Adipocyte

Fat tissue

Fig. 1.17 Leptin feedback loop. (Modified with permission from Sørensen, T.I.A. *et al.* 1996. *British Medical Journal* 313, 953–954.)

the hypothalamo–pituitary–adrenal axis could contribute to whole-body insulin resistance (see Section 2.6.1). Elevated interleukin-6 levels have been identified as a risk factor for type 2 diabetes in women. C-reactive protein, an acute phase reactant, has also been shown to predict type 2 diabetes.

Leptin

The cloning of the *ob*-gene and identification of its product, leptin in 1994 opened a new era of research into obesity. Leptin is a 167 amino acid protein synthesized and secreted by adipocytes which provides a feedback signal from adipose tissue to receptors in the hypothalamus (Fig. 1.17). Visceral adipocytes, which are considered in more detail in

Leptin signals information about adipose tissue stores to the hypothalamus

Section 2, appear to produce less leptin than their subcutaneous counterparts.

Leptin traverses the blood–brain barrier to inhibit the synthesis of neuropeptide Y, a tyrosine-containing peptide with powerful stimulatory effects on appetite. High leptin levels, indicative of an excessive adipose tissue mass, also lead to increased thermogenesis (neuropeptide Y also inhibits the activity of thermogenic brown adipose tissue in the rat). These effects serve to limit further weight gain. Mutant animal models in which leptin (*ob/ob* mouse) or its hypothalamic receptor (*db/db* mouse, *fa/fa* rat) are absent are associated with obesity and insulin resistance. However, circulating leptin concentrations are elevated in most obese humans implying defective signalling, i.e. cellular resistance to leptin, rather than deficiency of the protein.

Elevated plasma leptin concentrations are implicated in the aetiology of obesity-associated insulin resistance

Plasma leptin concentrations correlate with hyperinsulinaemia independently of body mass index. Hyperleptinaemia has been implicated in causing obesity-associated insulin resistance via effects on insulin signalling. Conversely, animal studies indicate that insulin may directly affect leptin concentrations. Leptin is also produced by the placenta and a role for leptin in female reproductive function is emerging.

Resistin

A novel adipocyte-derived hormone—resistin—was described in 2001 by Steppan *et al.* The peptide was discovered during a search for genes that are activated during adipocyte differentiation. Circulating levels of resistin are elevated in diet-induced and genetic murine models of obesity and type 2 diabetes. Immunoneutralization of resistin lowers blood glucose and improves insulin action whereas administration of the hormone impairs glucose tolerance and insulin action in normal mice. Data in humans is scanty but suggests that omental expression of resistin mRNA is higher than in subcutaneous adipocytes from other sites. The physiological role of human resistin (which has ~50% homology with murine resistin) remains to be elucidated. The discovery of adipocytokines such as resistin has helped to dispel the traditional view of fat as being a passive depot for triglycerides. Adipose tissue is now regarded as a metabolically active endocrine organ.

Adiponectin

Adiponectin is another recently identified adipocyte-derived hormone belonging to the collectin family Levels of adiponectin are reduced in human obesity and can be increased by treatment with thiazolidinediones (see Section 3.2.2.). Adiponectin promotes fatty acid oxidation in muscle thereby providing a potential link between obesity and impaired insulin action in myocytes. Adiponectin is also credited with anti-atherogenic properties.

Defective insulin pulsatility

Insulin is normally secreted by the β-cells in regular ~13-min pulses. Defective pulsatility has been identified as an early abnormality in studies in glucose-intolerant subjects and first-degree relatives of patients with type 2 diabetes. Experimental data demonstrate that some of the metabolic effects of insulin are enhanced when the hormone is delivered in pulses rather than as a continuous infusion. These observations raise the possibility that insulin action in target tissues might be impaired as a consequence of impaired endogenous pulsatility.

Defective insulin pulsatility is an early defect in glucose intolerance

Tissue enzyme activities

Impaired activities of key enzymes involved in tissue glucose metabolism have been identified in patients with obesity and type 2 diabetes. However, determining whether these are primary defects or consequences of the metabolic derangements has been problematic. Recent evidence favours the latter explanation, at least for glycogen synthesis in type 2 diabetes. However, animal studies show that the expression of key enzymes in carbohydrate metabolism may be modulated by exposure to glucocorticoids *in utero*. A key regulatory enzyme in the gluconeogenesis pathway (the formation of glucose from 3-carbon intermediates) —phosphoenolpyruvate carboxykinase—can be permanently increased in rats by dexamethasone treatment during the last trimester of pregnancy. Thus, excessive fetal glucocorticoid exposure *in utero* may lead to altered metabolic pathways in adult life. This also holds for low-protein diets

Impaired expression and activity of enzymes involved in carbohydrate metabolism are of uncertain significance

Glucocorticoid exposure in utero may lead to altered metabolic pathways in adult life

during gestation, which alter the tissue ratio of phosphoenolpyruvate carboxykinase : glucokinase. These are examples of the concept of 'metabolic programming' which is currently attracting considerable attention.

1.6.3 Fetal origins hypothesis

Metabolic programming is central to the fetal origins hypothesis advanced by Professor David Barker in Southampton, UK. This hypothesis links intrauterine growth retardation with insulin resistance and other major risk factors for cardiovascular disease in adults. According to the hypothesis:

'Coronary heart disease is associated with specific patterns of disproportionate fetal growth that results from fetal undernutrition in middle to later gestation.'

Barker developed his hypothesis to explain observations in a cohort from an English population that low birth weight during the early decades of the 20th century was associated with increased risk of coronary heart disease in adulthood. From this and other studies Barker *et al.* hypothesized that fetal undernutrition led to the following risk factors for coronary heart disease in adults.

- Insulin resistance.
- Islet β-cell dysfunction.
- Impaired glucose tolerance.
- Type 2 diabetes.
- Hypertension.
- Dyslipidaemia.
- Hyperfibrinogenemia.

Barker found that the risk of glucose intolerance or type 2 diabetes in middle-aged men (59–70 years) in the English cohort was inversely associated with birth weight. The odds ratio (adjusted for body mass index) for glucose intolerance ranged from 1.0 for birth weight > 4.3 kg to 6.6 for birth weight < 2.5 kg (Table 1.4).

These observations have been replicated in other populations from the USA and Sweden. Furthermore, a high placental weight and low body weight at age 12 months are also associated with hypertension and risk of coronary death, respectively. Recent data have countered the suggestion that confounding factors may have been responsible

Table 1.4 Odds ratios (adjusted for body mass index) for glucose intolerance (120 min glucose > 7.8 mmol/L) and type 2 diabetes in men aged 59–70 years. (From Hales, C.N. *et al.* 1991. *British Medical Journal* **303**, 1019–1022.)

Birth weight (g)	Total *n*	Impaired glucose tolerance or type 2 diabetes (%)	Odds ratio
< 2500	20	40	6.6
2540–2950	47	34	4.8
2990–3410	104	31	4.6
3450–3860	117	22	2.6
3900–4310	54	13	1.4
> 4310	28	14	1.0
Total	370	25	χ^2 for trend = 15.4*

* $P < 0.001$.

for observations that adult hypertension is more common in the lower birth-weight sibling in twin studies.

Postulated mechanisms of fetal programming

Barker proposes that intrauterine undernutrition at critical periods of fetal growth may lead to permanent structural and metabolic alterations which predispose to coronary heart disease. These result from compensatory mechanisms which serve to divert nutrients preferentially to the developing central nervous system. In turn, these lead to skeletal underdevelopment, a reduced β-cell mass and tissue vascular abnormalities. Animal studies of fetal undernutrition provide support for the fetal origins hypothesis which has provided a challenge to the genetic explanation for the well-recognized familial risk of type 2 diabetes.

The fetal origins hypothesis proposes that intrauterine undernutrition may lead to permanent structural and metabolic alterations

Additional observations from Barker's UK studies include the following.

• *Effect of obesity.* The development of obesity in subjects with the lowest birth weights was associated with the highest risk of glucose intolerance. A subsequent twin study showed that the lower birth-weight twin was more likely to develop type 2 diabetes as an adult. Islet β-cell dysfunction—increased circulating concentrations of proinsulin-like molecules—in middle-aged subjects of low birth weight has also been found.

• *Insulin resistance.* An association between decreased insulin sensitivity in adulthood, determined by the insulin tolerance test, and low ponderal index (a measure of thinness at birth) was observed in an English cohort for whom detailed birth records were available.

• *Decreased muscle glycolysis.* In another study of this cohort, ^{31}P magnetic spectroscopy showed a relationship between low ponderal index and lower lactate and adenosine triphosphate generation in skeletal muscle. Thus, there is evidence linking impaired fetal growth with alterations in insulin sensitivity and muscle metabolism in adults.

Thrifty phenotype hypothesis

This term was coined by Barker and Hales to distinguish metabolically programmed from inherited tissue structure and function which is encompassed in Neel's original 'thrifty genotype' hypothesis (see Section 2.5.5). Other investigators, notably Reaven, have suggested that insulin resistance may have a protective role in times of food deprivation by reducing the rate of muscle glucose utilization. This, in turn, would conserve glucose for obligate central nervous system requirements. Ultimately, skeletal muscle proteolysis, which would otherwise provide an alternative source of gluconeogenic precursors, would also be reduced and structural protein would thereby be conserved.

A thrifty phenotype may confer a survival advantage in periods of famine

Hypothalamo–pituitary–adrenal axis overactivity

Abnormalities in the hypothalamo–pituitary–adrenal axis have emerged as a potential cause or contributor to insulin resistance related to low birth weight. Cross-sectional studies in adults have shown an inverse relation between plasma cortisol concentrations and birth weight. Activation of the hypothalamo–pituitary–adrenal axis has also been observed in stimulation studies.

Activation of the hypothalamo–pituitary–adrenal axis is associated with low birth weight

Fetal insulin hypothesis

Other investigators have offered alternative genetic explanations that appear to be consistent with Barker's observations. Hattersley *et al.* in Exeter, UK, have produced

Genetically
determined defects
in fetal insulin
secretion can also
result in reduced
birth weight

evidence supporting an effect of monogenic defects in maternal and fetal insulin secretion (i.e. uncommon mutations in the glucose-sensing β-cell enzyme glucokinase, see Section 2.5.5) which can also produce a low birth weight phenotype. Other rare congenital conditions associated with decreased or absent fetal insulin secretion and low birth weight include:

• Pancreatic agenesis.

• Transient neonatal diabetes.

Conversely, nesidioblastosis—a rare condition resulting from homozygous mutations causing constitutive activation of the β-cell sulphonylurea receptor—is associated with birth weights which are usually > 90th percentile. This appears to be consistent with the anabolic actions of insulin (see Section 1.2.1). Much more common is the well-recognized association between maternal third trimester hyperglycaemia and macrosomia. This is held to be a consequence of the growth-promoting consequences of fetal hyperinsulinaemia which in turn results from β-cell stimulation by increased transfer of nutrients across the placenta. In the Pima Indians of Arizona, who have the highest recorded prevalence of type 2 diabetes, the risk of adult diabetes is related both to low and high birth weight in a bimodal relationship. The latter observation provides support for an adverse effect of intrauterine overnutrition with diabetes. However, the exceptionally high frequencies of obesity and diabetes in this population may confound the relationship between genes and intrauterine environment. In addition, in a white population a variation in the regulatory minisatellite 5′ to the insulin gene, which is a polymorphism associated with type 2 diabetes, has also been shown to influence fetal growth. Theoretically, impaired insulin secretion, insulin resistance, fetal growth and metabolism in adult life might be united through this or other mechanisms.

1.7 Further reading

American Diabetes Association (1998) Consensus development conference on insulin resistance. *Diabetes Care* 21, 310–314.

Andrews, R.C. & Walker, B.R. (1999) Glucocorticoids and insulin resistance: old hormone, new targets. *Clinical Science* 96, 513–523.

Barker, D.J. (1995) Intrauterine programming of adult disease. *Molecular Medicine Today* 1, 418–423.

Björntorp, P., Holm, G. & Rosmond, R. (1999) Hypothalamic arousal, insulin resistance and type 2 diabetes mellitus. *Diabetic Medicine* 16, 373–383.

Caro, J.F., Sinha, M.K., Kolaczynski, J.W., Zhang, P.L. & Considine, R.V. (1996) Leptin: the tale of an obesity gene. *Diabetes* 45, 1355–1462.

Ferrannini, E., Haffner, S.M., Mitchell, B.D. & Stern, M.P. (1991) Hyperinsulinaemia: the key feature of a cardiovascular and metabolic syndrome. *Diabetologia* 34, 416–422.

Groop, L.C., Widén, E. & Ferrannini, E. (1993) Insulin resistance and insulin deficiency in the pathogenesis of type 2 (non-insulin-dependent) diabetes mellitus: errors of metabolism or of methods? *Diabetologia* 36, 1326–1331.

Hales, C.N. & Barker, D.J. (1992) Type 2 (non-insulin-dependent) diabetes mellitus: the thrifty phenotype hypothesis. *Diabetologia* 35, 595–601.

Hattersley, A.T. & Tooke, J.E. (1999) The fetal insulin hypothesis: an alternative explanation of the association of low birthweight with diabetes and vascular disease. *Lancet* 353, 1789–1792.

Himsworth, H.P. (1936) Diabetes mellitus: a differentiation into insulin-sensitive and insulin-insensitive types. *Lancet* 1, 127–130.

Kahn, C.R. (1978) Insulin resistance, insulin insensitivity and insulin unresponsiveness: a necessary distinction. *Metabolism* 27, 1893–1902.

Krentz, A.J. (1996) Insulin resistance. *British Medical Journal* 313, 1385–1389.

Krentz, A.J. & Nattrass, M. (1996) Insulin resistance: a multifaceted metabolic syndrome. Insights gained using a low-dose insulin infusion technique. *Diabetic Medicine* 13, 30–39.

Krook, A. & O'Rahilly, S. (1996) Mutant insulin receptors in syndromes of insulin resistance. *Baillière's Clinical Endocrinology and Metabolism* 10, 97–122.

Le Roith, D. & Zick, Y. (2001) Recent advances in our understanding of insulin action and insulin resistance. *Diabetes Care* 24, 588–597.

Mari, A., Pacini, G., Murphy, E., Ludvik, B. & Nolan, J.J. (2001) A model-based method for assessing insulin sensitivity from the oral glucose tolerance test. *Diabetes Care* 24, 539–548.

Mauriege, P. & Bouchard, C. (1996) Trp64Arg mutation in β_3-adrenoceptor gene of doubtful significance for obesity and insulin resistance. *Lancet* 348, 698–699.

McClain, D.A. & Crook, E.D. (1996) Hexosamines and insulin resistance. *Diabetes* 45, 1003–1009.

Moller, D. (ed.) (1993) *Insulin Resistance*, John Wiley, Chichester.

Moller, D.E. & Flier, J.S. (1991) Insulin resistance—mechanisms, syndromes, and implications. *New England Journal of Medicine* **325**, 938–948.

Nattrass, M. & Dodds, K.E. (1987) Interpretation of insulin radioreceptor assays. *Annals of Clinical Biochemistry* **24**, 13–21.

Pedersen, O. (1999) Genetics of insulin resistance. *Experimental and Clinical Endocrinology and Diabetes* **107**, 113–118.

Perry, C., Sattar, N. & Petrie, J. (2001) Adipose tissue: passive sump or active pump? *British Journal of Diabetes and Vascular Disease* **1**, 110–114.

Phillips, D.I.W. (1996) Insulin resistance as a programmed response to fetal undernutrition. *Diabetologia* **39**, 1119–1122.

Randle, P.J., Garland, P.B., Hales, C.N. & Newsholme, E.A. (1963) The glucose–fatty-acid cycle: its role in insulin insensitivity and the metabolic disturbances of diabetes mellitus. *Lancet* **1**, 785–789.

Reaven, G.M. (1988) Role of insulin resistance in human disease. *Diabetes* **37**, 1595–1607.

Reaven, G.M. (1998) Hypothesis: muscle insulin resistance is the ('not-so') thrifty genotype. *Diabetologia* **41**, 482–484.

Scheen, A.J., Paquot, N., Castillo, M.J. & Lefèbvre, P.J. (1994) How to measure insulin action *in vivo*. *Diabetes/Metabolism Reviews* **2**, 151–188.

Seckl, J.R. (1998) Physiologic programming of the fetus. *Clinical Perinatology* **25**, 939–964.

Shepherd, P.R. & Kahn, B.B. (1999) Glucose transporters and insulin action. Implications for insulin resistance and diabetes mellitus. *New England Journal of Medicine* **341**, 248–257.

Shulman, G.I. (2000) Cellular mechanisms of insulin resistance. *Journal of Clinical Investigation* **106**, 171–176.

Stears, A.J. & Byrne, C.D. (2001) Adipocyte metabolism and the metabolic syndrome. *Diabetes, Obesity, Metabolism* **3**, 129–142.

Steppan, C.M., Bailey, S.T. & Bhat, S. *et al.* (2001) The hormone resistin links obesity to diabetes. *Nature* **409**, 307–312.

Stumvoll, M., Meyer, C., Mitrakou, A., Nadkarni, V. & Gerich, J.E. (1997) Renal glucose production and utilization: new aspects in humans. *Diabetologia* **40**, 749–757.

Temple, R., Clark, P.M.S. & Hales, C.N. (1992) Measurement of insulin secretion in type 2 diabetes: problems and pitfalls. *Diabetic Medicine* **9**, 503–512.

Unger, R.H. (1995) Lipotoxicity in the pathogenesis of obesity-dependent NIDDM. *Diabetes* **44**, 863–870.

Unger, R.H. & Grundy, S. (1985) Hyperglycaemia as an inducer as well as a consequence of impaired islet cell function and insulin resistance: implications for the management of diabetes. *Diabetologia* **28**, 119–121.

2 Insulin resistance in clinical medicine

2.1 Clinical features

Common inherited or acquired disorders

The clinical relevance of insulin resistance is uncertain in many conditions

Many common inherited or acquired disorders in humans are associated with insulin resistance. In some, e.g. impaired glucose tolerance or type 2 diabetes, the insulin resistance is almost universal and is regarded as a major factor in the aetiology of the disorder. In others, e.g. polycystic ovary disease, insulin resistance is emerging as an important target for therapeutic intervention. However, for many of the conditions in which impaired insulin action has been documented the relevance of the metabolic defect to aetiology and ultimately to treatment remains far less clear.

The latter group includes essential hypertension, heart failure and chronic renal failure. Failure to control for factors such as decreased physical activity and fitness in metabolic studies of these debilitating conditions may in part explain some of this uncertainty. Importantly, insulin resistance is asymptomatic in the absence of metabolic decompensation, i.e. diabetes mellitus, or other features, e.g. hyperandrogenism in women.

Insulin resistance per se is asymptomatic

As direct measurement of insulin sensitivity is problematic (see Section 1.5), insulin resistance is usually inferred in clinical practice from associated clinical or biochemical features, such as obesity or type 2 diabetes. A number of uncommon or rare inherited syndromes with specific and readily identifiable phenotypes are associated with insulin resistance, e.g. myotonic dystrophy. Hyper-secretory endocrinopathies (see Section 2.6.2), such as Cushing's syndrome and acromegaly, will often be accompanied by significant insulin resistance in addition to characteristic features of the particular syndrome. More specific physical signs suggestive of pathological degrees of insulin resistance include the following:

• *Acanthosis nigricans*. This hyperkeratotic papillomatous condition is recognized by pigmented plaques, usually most evident on the axillae, antecubital fossae, the nape of the neck and other skin folds. Multiple skin tags (acrochordons) may also be present in affected individuals. Acanthosis is almost universal in patients with congenital syndromes of severe insulin resistance (see Section 2.4). It may also be found in patients with less severe acquired forms of insulin resistance, such as that associated with obesity, endocrinopathies and polycystic ovary syndrome (see Section 2.5.12). Racial differences in the prevalence of acanthosis nigricans are recognised; in a US study approximately 10% of black or hispanic school children were found to have evidence of this marker. The molecular mechanisms responsible for acanthosis remain undetermined. Since insulin can cross-react with mitogenic insulin-like growth factor-1 receptor, stimulation by the latter by hyperinsulinaeminia has been proposed. However, the evidence does not provide convincing support for this theory. For disfiguring acanthosis, 5% salicylic acid cream is recommended.

Acanthosis nigricans is a cutaneous marker for insulin resistance

• *Hyperandrogenism.* Cutaneous stigmata of ovarian hyperandrogenism include hirsutism and acne vulgaris, both of which are prominent symptoms in women with polycystic ovary syndrome. Chronic anovulation with menstrual irregularity or secondary amenorrhoea is common (see Section 2.5.12). HAIR-AN syndrome refers to the constellation of hyperandrogenism, insulin resistance and acanthosis nigricans.

• *Acromegaloid features.* Acral hypertrophy (with muscle cramps) and other acromegaloid features (enlargement of pinnae, macroglossia) are occasionally encountered in patients with severe insulin resistance and very high plasma insulin levels. Circulating growth hormone and insulin-like growth factor-1 concentrations are normal. As for acanthosis, the mechanism is unexplained. It has been suggested that insulin resistance in glucose disposal may not always be reflected in insulin resistance in other metabolic pathways. Thus, other anabolic and mitogenic pathways of insulin (Table 1.1) might be stimulated by compensatory hyperinsulinaemia. This hypothesis is frequently referred to as tissue selective insulin resistance. However, rather than implying an all-or-nothing effect, differences in dose–response relationships between metabolic and mitogenic pathways could, at least in theory, result in divergent tissue actions.

• *Precocious pseudo-puberty.* In conjunction with phallic enlargement, these are variable features of some congenital severe insulin-resistance syndromes.

• *Growth retardation.* Intrauterine growth retardation with low birth weight is another variable feature of syndromes associated with severe insulin resistance. Profound impairment of insulin action within the developing fetus is consistent with the fetal insulin hypothesis (see Section 1.6.3), albeit an extreme manifestation.

• *Lipodystrophy.* Congenital and acquired lipodystrophic syndromes are discussed in Section 2.4.

2.2 Factors influencing insulin sensitivity

The many factors influencing insulin sensitivity must be taken into consideration when studies of human insulin action are carried out. Of these, body mass index and environmental factors are thought to account for approximately 30% of variance in insulin action. Other potential confounding variables, some of which may not be readily apparent in otherwise healthy subjects, have not always been excluded or matched for in case-control studies.

2.2.1 Normal variation in insulin action

There is a wide range of insulin sensitivity within otherwise healthy populations

Even when efforts are expended to minimize the impact of such factors, insulin sensitivity in the normal population still varies considerably between individuals at any specified body mass index (Fig. 2.1).

Data abound demonstrating the wide variability in insulin action in healthy individuals. For example, Reaven found there was a threefold variation in clamp-derived M-values (see Section 1.5.6) in subjects with normal glucose tolerance. The principal determinant of fasting plasma glucose concentrations under these circumstances is the degree of β-cell function. Accordingly, there is no clear relationship between fasting glucose concentrations and M-values among patients with glucose tolerance or type 2 diabetes.

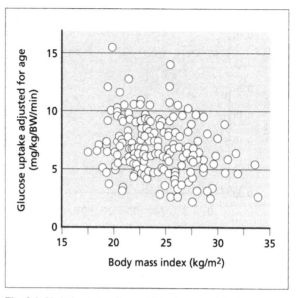

Fig. 2.1 Variation in insulin sensitivity (measured during euglycaemic clamps as a function of body mass index in 177 normoglycaemic Finnish subjects. (Redrawn with permission from Yki-Järvinen, H. 1995. *Diabetologia*; **38**, 1378–1388.)

Using a different technique—the intravenous glucose tolerance test (see Section 1.5.2)—Clausen *et al.* found a 10-fold variation in insulin sensitivity in a sample of healthy young adults (Fig. 2.2).

Figure 2.3 demonstrates that there is considerable overlap between insulin-mediated glucose disposal in patients with type 2 diabetes and matched non-diabetic control subjects when studied at physiological or pharmacological plasma insulin concentrations. Taken together, these studies demonstrate that insulin sensitivity is a continuous variable.

Although there is no consensus on a threshold for the definition of insulin resistance, when individuals in the lowest quantile of insulin sensitivity of Clausen's cohort were compared with the remainder of the sample, the former were found to be more obese and less glucose-tolerant. Moreover, the following cardiovascular risk factors were evident in the most insulin-resistant subgroup:

Insulin sensitivity is a continuous variable in healthy populations

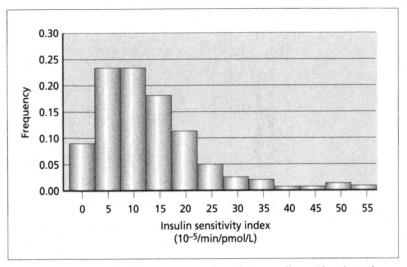

Fig. 2.2 Distribution of insulin sensitivity as estimated using a tolbutamide-enhanced intravenous glucose tolerance test in a population-based sample of 380 healthy white subjects aged 18–32 years. (Redrawn with permission from Clausen, J.O. *et al.* 1996. *Journal of Clinical Investigation* **98**, 1195–1209.)

- Higher fasting lipid concentrations.
- Higher blood pressure.
- Impaired fibrinolysis.

Similar associations in otherwise healthy subjects have been demonstrated in other studies of different populations (see Section 2.5.1). It has been proposed that non-obese subjects with metabolic features of the insulin resistance syndrome (see Section 2.5.1) may be at higher risk of type 2 diabetes and atherosclerotic disease in later life. Preventative measures might be appropriately targeted at such 'metabolically obese, normal weight' individuals. Other variables which require careful evaluation when performing metabolic studies include the following.

1 Modifiable factors:
- Body mass index.
- Regional distribution of adipose tissue.
- Aerobic fitness.
- Personal history of glucose intolerance.
- History of gestational diabetes.
- Phase of menstrual cycle.
- Hepatic and renal function.

Normal weight individuals with features of the insulin-resistance syndrome may be at increased risk of type 2 diabetes and cardiovascular disease

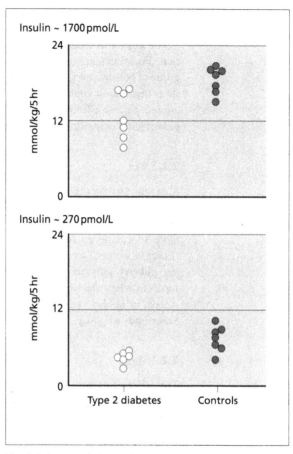

Fig. 2.3 Integrated glucose disposal over 5 h in patients with type 2 diabetes and healthy control subjects matched for age and sex. Divide by 6.0 to convert plasma insulin concentrations to mU/L. (Data with permission from Butler, P.C. *et al.* 1990. *Diabetes* **39**, 1373–1380.)

- Relevant medication, e.g. β-adrenergic blockers.
- Smoking habits.
- Habitual alcohol consumption.
- Plasma lipids, e.g. inherited dyslipidaemias.
- Chronic disorders, e.g. inflammatory disease, neoplasia.
- Recent acute illness.

2 Non-modifiable factors:
  - Sex.
  - Age.

- Family history of type 2 diabetes.
- Congenital syndromes associated with insulin resistance.

The impact of lifestyle factors merits further investigation. For example, an intriguing recent study in a small group of healthy young adults suggested that even minimal sleep deprivation could impair glucose tolerance (via decreased glucose effectiveness; Section 1.5.4) and increase plasma levels of insulin-antagonistic hormones.

2.2.2 Sex

Men and women normally have approximately equal insulin sensitivity, if factors such as differences in body composition (in general, women have approximately 10% more subcutaneous adipose tissue) and aerobic capacity (lower in women) are taken into account. However, during puberty girls are more insulin-resistant than boys. Lipolysis is less well suppressed in women with an android pattern of obesity (see Section 2.5.3) than in those with lower-body adiposity.

2.2.3 Age

The effect of ageing on insulin sensitivity is disputed

The effect of ageing, *per se*, on insulin sensitivity is disputed. However, glucose tolerance tends to deteriorate with advancing age and increasing insulin resistance has been implicated in some cross-sectional studies. The proportion of fat in central depots tends to increase in middle age (see Section 2.5.3). Declining β-cell function is also likely to be important. A recent analysis of pooled glucose clamp data from several European centres did not provide support for decreasing insulin sensitivity with age.

2.2.4 Physical exercise

Key points:
- Regular physical exercise improves insulin sensitivity.
- Insulin sensitivity rapidly declines with immobilization.

These well-established effects have frequently been ignored or under-appreciated in studies of insulin action in humans.

Physical exercise improves insulin action

Maximal oxygen uptake (Vo_{2max})—a measure of exercise capacity—may be partially under genetic control. Insulin-resistant relatives with type 2 diabetes and subjects with central obesity have low Vo_{2max} levels. These are accompanied by vascular changes in skeletal muscle:

- Lower capillary density.
- Greater white : red fibre ratio, i.e. fewer insulin-sensitive fibres.

However, whether these changes, which indicate decreased aerobic capacity, reflect genetics or differences in physical activity status is unclear. Nonetheless, physical training appears to be beneficial particularly in countering the metabolic defects associated with visceral adiposity (see Section 2.5.3).

Physical inactivity

The potential health benefits of regular physical activity remain rather neglected. Inactive adults have approximately twice the risk of premature death and serious medical illness as active individuals; the relative risk associated with a sedentary lifestyle being similar to that associated with hypertension or hypercholesterolaemia. Such observations are of particular relevance to patients with established type 2 diabetes (see Section 2.5.5). Data from the Nurses' Health Study suggest an independent protective role against the development of type 2 diabetes from regular exercise; even habitual brisk walking is effective in reducing the risk.

The beneficial effects of physical exercise and its role in the management of obesity and type 2 diabetes are discussed in more detail in Section 3. Recent data suggests that physical fitness may be protective even in obese subjects.

A sedentary lifestyle is a major risk factor for coronary heart disease

Regular brisk walking can protect against type 2 diabetes

Physiology of acute exercise

The breakdown of glycogen provides the initial energy for exercising skeletal muscle. Glycogen is rapidly depleted and the demand for glucose is matched by an increase in hepatic glucose production. During prolonged exercise mobilization of fatty acids from adipose tissue increases substantially. This provides the major source of energy for continuing muscular contraction and may contribute to the acute insulin resistance which follows a marathon run.

Prolonged exercise is associated with an increase in insulin resistance

These metabolic actions result primarily from rapid changes in circulating levels of insulin and counter-regulatory hormones, notably catecholamines. The decline in plasma insulin levels allows mobilization of glucose from the liver. Lowered endogenous insulin secretion also permits lipolysis to accelerate; this is augmented by the lipolytic action of the sympatho–adrenal system. Thus, there is a close match of substrate provision to consumption by myocytes.

Exercise in diabetic patients

For diabetic patients treated with exogenous insulin, and to a lesser extent those treated with sulphonylureas, the inability to acutely lower plasma insulin levels requires strategies to enable exercise to continue without the rapid development of hypoglycaemia. These include reducing insulin doses before exercise and increasing oral carbohydrate intake. Late hypoglycaemia, occurring many hours after acute exercise, is a recognized hazard.

Exercise-induced hypoglycaemia is a hazard for insulin-treated diabetics

2.2.5 Tobacco

Insulin sensitivity

Tobacco use is increasing in many developing countries in which the incidence of obesity and type 2 diabetes is also rising. Several studies have suggested that habitual cigarette smoking is associated with hyperinsulinaemia, glucose intolerance and reduced insulin sensitivity as measured with quantitative techniques. Impaired insulin-mediated suppression of lipolysis has also been demonstrated. However, some epidemiological data does not support an association between smoking and hyperinsulinaemia.

Cigarette smoking is associated with reduced insulin sensitivity

Smoking acutely stimulates the sympatho–adrenal system and increases the circulating levels of counter-regulatory hormones (see Section 2.6.1). Abnormalities in plasma lipoproteins are also well recognized in habitual smokers. However, controlling for potential confounding factors, such as differences in aerobic capacity, body composition (smokers tend to have more abdominal fat), dietary differences, etc., presents difficulties in clinical studies.

Effect of smoking cessation

Smoking cessation is associated with improved insulin sensitivity. This effect appears to exceed the converse effect of any weight gain. Limited data suggest that nicotine replacement may also cause insulin resistance. The deleterious effects of tobacco are considered in more detail in Section 3.1.4.

2.2.6 Alcohol

Moderate habitual consumption of alcohol is associated with reduced plasma insulin concentrations in a dose-dependent fashion. However, excessive alcohol leads to elevated blood pressure and may aggravate hypertriglyceridaemia. Alcohol and the insulin-resistance syndrome are discussed in more detail in Section 3.1.3.

2.3 Physiological states of insulin resistance

Reduced insulin sensitivity is observed in certain physiological situations, notably in women during:

* Puberty.
* The second and third trimesters of pregnancy.
* The menopause.

Compensatory insulin secretion usually ensures that the insulin resistance associated with puberty or pregnancy remains subclinical. However, this physiological insulin resistance may have important implications for patients with diabetes or limited β-cell reserves.

Puberty, pregnancy and phase of menstrual cycle may influence insulin sensitivity

2.3.1 Puberty

Growth hormone is the principal cause of insulin resistance in puberty

Puberty is associated with transient insulin resistance. Changes in body composition may contribute but the main cause of the decrease in insulin sensitivity is thought to be increased growth hormone secretion.

Insulin resistance in adolescents correlates with circulating insulin-like growth factor-1 concentrations. In children with pre-existing diabetes, increased insulin requirements necessitate larger doses of insulin. Thus, the daily insulin

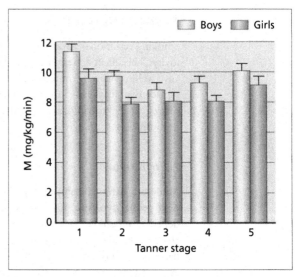

Fig. 2.4 Insulin resistance (*M*-value) by Tanner stage and sex, adjusted for body mass index. The cohort of 159 girls was more insulin resistant than the cohort of 198 boys (*P* < 0.0001). Girls appeared to be more insulin resistant than boys at each Tanner stage. (Redrawn with permission from Moran, A. *et al.* 1999. *Diabetes* **48**, 2039–2044.)

Insulin
requirements
increase
substantially
during adolescence
in patients with
type 1 diabetes

dose required by children with type 1 diabetes increases from approximately 0.5 to > 1.0 U/kg with the onset of puberty. In a recently published study of euglycaemic clamp studies performed in US children aged 10–14 years the following observations were presented (Fig. 2.4):

• Insulin resistance (*M*-value) increased at the onset of puberty.

• Peak insulin resistance occurred at Tanner stage 3.

• Girls were more insulin-resistant than boys.

• Insulin resistance was strongly related to measures of overall and regional adiposity.

• Differences in adiposity did not, however, entirely explain the insulin resistance of puberty.

• White boys were more insulin resistant than black boys, there being no differences between girls.

2.3.2 Pregnancy

Pregnancy is associated with alterations in the regulation of

Pregnancy is a physiological state of insulin resistance

glucose metabolism caused by the actions of human placental lactogen and progesterone; these hormones antagonize the actions of insulin, leading to a state of relative insulin resistance as pregnancy progresses. Lipolysis is also accelerated, despite hyperinsulinaemia. Accordingly, pregnancy is regarded as a state of accelerated ketosis.

In women with normal β-cell function, the insulin resistance associated with pregnancy is compensated for by increased insulin secretion. However, the additional insulin resistance means that women with pre-existing type 1 diabetes need higher doses of insulin as pregnancy progresses. Women with type 2 diabetes treated with diet or tablets often require insulin treatment during pregnancy. Glucose intolerance or diabetes may be precipitated in predisposed women who previously had normal glucose tolerance. Although glucose tolerance usually normalizes postpartum, women who develop gestational diabetes are at considerably increased risk of developing permanent type 2 diabetes in the longer term. The risk varies according to ethnicity, amongst other factors. The metabolic changes associated with pregnancy include the following.

• *First trimester.* Fasting glucose concentrations decline modestly in non-diabetic women reaching a nadir at approximately 12 weeks. The renal clearance of glucose is increased, reflecting an increase in glomerular filtration rate (in the absence of any change in maximal reabsorption via the renal tubules). Post-prandial glucose levels, by contrast, tend to rise whereas plasma insulin concentrations are unchanged. Effects on insulin requirements may also be influenced by pregnancy-associated nausea and vomiting.

• *Second and third trimesters.* The regulatory effects of insulin on carbohydrate and fat metabolism become impaired, i.e. a state of relative insulin resistance develops. It has been hypothesized that these metabolic changes facilitate transfer of maternal nutrients to the fetus. In insulin-treated women, insulin requirements may increase markedly between weeks 28 and 32 of gestation; insulin requirements may decline to some extent after 35 weeks.

Insulin requirements in diabetic women rapidly return to prepregnancy levels postpartum

• *Parturition.* During delivery, with separation of the placenta, insulin requirements fall very rapidly to prepregnancy levels.

Use of ritodrine
and dexamethasone
for premature
labour induces
severe acute insulin
resistance

Use of β-adrenergic agonists, such as ritodrine in conjunction with high-dose corticosteroids (to suppress premature labour and accelerate fetal lung maturity, respectively), may induce acute severe insulin resistance. In diabetic mothers this combination may necessitate high doses of intravenous insulin to avert metabolic decompensation. The metabolic effects of hormonal contraceptive preparations are considered in Section 2.8.

2.3.3 Menstrual cycle

A high proportion of insulin-treated diabetic females of reproductive age report fluctuating insulin requirements in relation to their menstrual cycle. In some, insulin requirements appear to be lowest between days 7 and 21 of the cycle, rising gradually until the onset of menstruation. The cause of this variability in insulin requirements, which is rarely marked, is uncertain. Glucose clamp studies have produced inconsistent results, those in non-diabetic women generally showing no difference between the follicular and luteal phases of the cycle.

The impact of the
menstrual cycle on
insulin sensitivity is
unclear

By contrast, at least one study demonstrated impaired glucose uptake in a small group of women with type 1 diabetes whose insulin requirements were higher in the luteal phase. Of more relevance clinically is the chronic anovulation and oligo- or amenorrhoea associated with polycystic ovary syndrome (see Section 2.5.12).

2.3.4 The menopause

Animal studies indicate that loss of oestrogen secretion induces a state of insulin resistance which can be reversed by replacement therapy. Oestrogen deficiency is accompanied by changes in body composition, including a shift towards a more androgenic (central) distribution of adipose tissue. Studies in postmenopausal women suggest a progressive decline in tissue insulin sensitivity (Fig. 2.5) which is accompanied by increased endogenous insulin secretion. Impaired endogenous insulin responses have also been linked to oestrogen deficiency.

Oestrogen
deficiency is
associated with
relative insulin
resistance

It not known whether decreasing insulin sensitivity contributes directly to the increased risk of cardiovascular

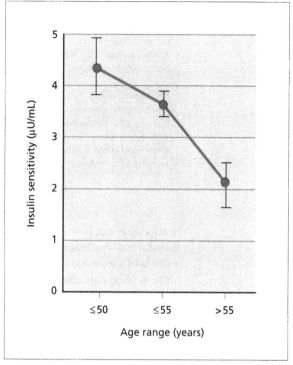

Fig. 2.5 Effect of age on insulin sensitivity in non-obese postmenopausal women. (Adapted with permission from Walton, C. *et al.* 1993. *European Journal of Clinical Investigation* **23**, 466–473.)

disease that accompanies the menopause. However, adverse effects on circulating lipoproteins are well documented. These effects may be particularly important in women with type 2 diabetes who tend to have hypertriglycaeridaemia and low high density lipoprotein (HDL)-cholesterol concentrations. The metabolic effects of oestrogen replacement therapy are discussed in Section 2.8.

2.4 Severe insulin-resistance syndromes

Rare genetic or acquired syndromes of severe insulin resistance offer insights into the importance of impaired insulin action to human disease. These syndromes are usually manifested as dramatic disturbances of carbohydrate

Table 2.1 Syndromes associated with severe insulin resistance.

Insulin receptor mutations
Leprechaunism
Rabson–Mendenhall syndrome
Type A insulin resistance
Post-binding defects in insulin action
Lipodystrophy syndromes
Type C insulin resistance
Anti-insulin receptor antibodies
Type B insulin resistance

metabolism and, in the case of the genetic syndromes, of growth and development. Although rarely encountered outside of specialized centres, the scientfic importance of these syndromes justifies an appreciation of the major recognized defects (Table 2.1).

Insulin receptor mutations

More than 50 mutations of the insulin receptor have been described (see Section 1.6.1). The severity of the insulin resistance in such syndromes is reflected by massive hyperinsulinaemia; plasma insulin concentrations may be as much as 100-times greater than normal. Glucose tolerance may be well preserved but there may be glucose intolerance progressing to type 2 diabetes. Severe ketoacidosis is not usually a feature.

Leprechaunism

Patients with this syndrome have one of the most profound forms of insulin resistance. The phenotype includes intrauterine growth retardation, acanthosis nigricans and hyperandrogenism with hirsutism; postprandial hyperglycaemia with fasting hypoglycaemia may occur. Survival beyond the first few years of life is unusual. Affected individuals are most often compound heterozygotes for missense or non-sense mutations of the insulin receptor gene. Decreased receptor affinity, binding or tyrosine kinase activity have been reported.

Rabson–Mendenhall syndrome

Specific phenotypic features of this syndrome include abnormal dentition, nail dystrophy, pineal hyperplasia and precocious pseudopuberty. Partial responses to insulin-like growth factor-1 have been described. Survival into the second or third decade has been reported. Ketoacidosis has occasionally been described.

Other inherited and acquired syndromes of severe insulin resistance

Lipodystrophic diabetes

These may be either congenital or acquired (Table 2.2). The acquired syndromes generally have their onset in early childhood. The principal phenotypic characteristic is partial or total absence of subcutaneous fat, variable degrees of insulin resistance and severe hyperlipidaemia (with risk of hypertriglyceridaemia-associated pancreatitis and accelerated atherosclerosis). Magnetic resonance imaging has identified minor adipose tissue in some sites, e.g. orbits, plantar surfaces of hands and feet. The paucity of adipose tissue leads to striking clinical appearances and ketosis-resistant diabetes. Intramuscular and hepatic triglyceride levels are increased. Cirrhosis is a feature of some forms. Complement activation and mesangioproliferative glomerulonephritis are features of cephalothoracic lipodystrophy

Table 2.2 The lipodystrophic syndromes.

Type	Associated features
Generalized syndromes	
Congential generalized lipoatrophy	Hypertriglyceridaemia Hyperandrogenism Cirrhosis
Acquired total lipoatrophy	Hyperlipidaemia Cirrhosis
Partial syndromes	
Face-sparing lipodystrophy	Hyperlipidaemia Hypertension
Cephalothoracic lipodystrophy	Glomerulonephritis Complement activation

(adipsin, secreted by adipocytes, is a component of the alternative complement pathway). Transplantation of adipose tissue into transgenic mouse models of lipoatrophy improves defects in carbohydrate and lipid metabolism. Mutations in the gene encoding the nuclear envelope protein lamin A/C (LMNA) are responsible for Dunnigan-type familial partial lipodystrophy (via unknown mechanisms).

Type A insulin resistance

The type A syndrome is caused by genetic defects in the insulin receptor. It is characterized by acanthosis nigricans, hyperinsulinaemia, glucose intolerance and variable degrees of hyperandrogenism and acromegaloidism. Neither obesity nor lipodystrophy are features. Virtually all reported cases have been in young women. Inheritance may be either autosomal dominant or autosomal recessive with variable penetrance.

Type B insulin resistance

This is an acquired syndrome in which IgG autoantibodies are directed against the insulin receptor. Variable blockade or stimulation of the receptor may occur. Black women over the age of 30 years comprise the majority of reported cases; acanthosis nigricans is common. Other features of autoimmune disease are common. Spontaneous remissions may occur. An autosomal recessive variant associated with ataxia telangiectasia caused by IgM antireceptor antibodies is recognized.

Type C insulin resistance

This is phenotypically similar to the type A syndrome. However, by definition, insulin receptors are normal and the defect in insulin action is located at a distal point.

Treatment of severe insulin-resistance syndromes

Treatment is directed towards the most prominent features in the particular patient.
• *Lifestyle measures.* The role of diet and exercise (see Section 3.1) are limited in the face of the severe impairment of insulin action.

Thiazolidinediones may be effective in some syndromes of severe insulin resistance

- *Insulin-sensitizing drugs.* These include metformin and thiazolidinediones (see Section 3.2.2). The use of such drugs appears logical and has met with some success; however, experience is limited. Moreover, these drugs are contraindicated in patients with lipodystrophy who have chronic liver disease (Table 2.2).
- *Sulphonylureas.* These drugs, which stimulate endogenous insulin secretion (see Section 3.2.3), should be used with caution in patients with syndromes such as Rabson–Mendenhall syndrome; catastrophic hypoglycaemia has been reported.
- *Exogenous insulin.* The development of overt diabetes poses therapeutic difficulties. Exogenous insulin requirements in excess of 1.5 U/kg daily may raise suspicion of one of these syndromes. However, in the absence of readily recognizable phenotypes, such as lipodystrophy, further metabolic assessment is indicated. Such investigations are most appropriately performed by specialist units. For insulin-treated patients, detailed testing may be required to exclude physical or psychological causes of apparent insulin resistance. Schade *et al.* developed a systematic approach to investigation and were able to exclude a putative 'subcutaneous insulin resistance syndrome' in a series of patients with glycaemic instability. However, for the patient with genuine severe insulin resistance, exogenous insulin requirements may prove to be enormous; doses amounting to thousands of units per day have been reported.
- *Insulin-like growth factor-1.* This hormone, which shares homology with insulin and can stimulate insulin receptors, been used experimentally in the type A syndrome and Rabson–Mendenhall syndrome (see Section 3.6).
- *Immunosuppressant drugs.* Measures directed against autoimmunity in the type B syndrome have met with variable success.
- *Future prospects.* Circumvention of receptor defects using antireceptor antibodies with agonist activity has been reported in an experimental setting.

2.5 Insulin resistance and cardiovascular risk

Insulin resistance is a recognized feature of a number of common disorders in humans. Frequently, these disorders cluster together in what is known as the insulin-resistance syndrome. This has a number of synonyms which are often loosely used interchangeably: Syndrome X, Reaven's syndrome and the metabolic syndrome.

The insulin-resistance syndrome has several synonyms

The insulin-resistance syndrome confers an increased risk of cardiovascular disease

Cardiac risk factors may be synergistic rather than additive when present in combination

Cardiovascular risk reduction involves treatment directed at all modifiable factors

Components of the insulin-resistance syndrome (see Section 2.5.1) are frequently present in combination. Whether insulin resistance is the fundamental metabolic defect which links these abnormalities remains uncertain. However, there is considerable epidemiological and experimental evidence that the insulin resistance syndrome confers an increased risk of cardiovascular disease. Importantly, the magnitude of the risk associated with a combination of factors can be greater than would be expected by simple addition, i.e. the effects are synergistic. Taking the example of type 2 diabetes, there is evidence from longitudinal studies that these metabolic risk factors worsen continuously across the spectrum of glucose intolerance and are present even before the diagnosis of type 2 diabetes. If a different perspective is taken, a substantial proportion of patients with essential hypertension have one or more additional components of the syndrome which contribute to their risk of cardiovascular events. There is an emerging consensus that reduction of cardiovascular risk demands attention to all modifiable factors.

Insulin and atherosclerosis

The earliest description of hyperinsulinaemia in patients with either coronary heart disease or peripheral vascular disease dates back to the 1960s. However, the nature of the association between insulin resistance and atherosclerosis remains uncertain. While a wealth of data from cross-sectional studies has demonstrated an association, no study has provided confirmation that insulin resistance is an independent predictor of atheroma. The relationship between insulin and atherogenesis remains controversial. Reaven has argued that insulin resistance, rather than compensatory hyper-insulinaemia, is a fundamental defect that increases the risk of cardiovascular disease through its associations with other risk factors. Direct effects of insulin on processes involved in atheroma formation have been demonstrated *in vitro*. However, the pharmacological concentrations of insulin employed in some studies is of dubious relevance to the usual situation in humans.

Recent clinical and experimental data contradict the view that exogenous insulin accelerates atherogenesis. None the less, concerns have long been expressed about the use of exogenous insulin in type 2 diabetes for fear of exacerbating atheroma. In the UK Prospective Diabetes Study (UKPDS, see Section 3.2), intensified therapy with either sulphonylureas or insulin was associated with a 16% *reduction* ($P = 0.052$) in myocardial infarction over 15 years (compared with diet). There was no evidence of a deleterious effect of intensified therapy on any of the macrovascular end-points studied. The Diabetes Control and Complications (DCCT) Trial also reported a nonsignificant trend towards a reduced incidence of macrovascular events in relatively young intensively treated patients with type 1 diabetes. Thus, both of these major randomized trials have provided evidence, albeit not conclusive, that intensive insulin therapy reduces rather than promotes atheroma.

Pharmacological insulin concentrations promote atherogenesis in experimental studies

In the UKPDS intensive therapy resulted in a 16% reduction in myocardial infarction

Coronary heart disease

Several studies have demonstrated the presence of hyperinsulinaemia or more direct evidence of insulin resistance in patients with coronary heart disease. However, small sample sizes, selection bias and the potential confounding effects of drugs and comorbidity detract to some extent from the reliability of the evidence. A number of long-term prospective studies (e.g. Busselton, Helsinki policemen, Paris policemen, Quebec, Kuopio) in non-diabetic individuals have also been reported. In brief, most of these studies provide support for the existence of an independent association between measures of fasting or stimulated hyperinsulinaemia and coronary heart disease. However, these observational studies do not establish a causal role for hyperinsulinaemia.

A recent meta-analysis concluded that insulin was a relatively weak risk-indicator for cardiovascular disease. The strength and nature of the association have differed between studies. Some studies (e.g. a recent analysis of the Multiple Risk Factor Intervention Trial (MRFIT) data)

Several long-term prospective studies have found an association between hyperinsulinaemia and coronary heart disease

have not confirmed an independent relationship between hyperinsulinaemia and coronary atheroma. When adjusted for a multiplicity of other risk factors, the associations are generally weakened. Interactions between insulin and other risk factors have been noted in some studies, e.g. with apolipoprotein E phenotype in the MRFIT cohort and apolipoprotein B in the Quebec study (Fig. 1.12). Finally, not all of these studies measured baseline levels of other important risk factors, e.g. HDL-cholesterol, that are closely related to insulin resistance.

Peripheral vascular disease

Evidence from several population-based cross-sectional studies also supports an association, again not necessarily causal, between hyperinsulinaemia or insulin resistance and peripheral vascular disease (assessed using a variety of techniques ranging from symptomatic intermittent claudication to ultrasonic measurement of carotid artery intimal thickness).

Peripheral vascular disease is associated with decreased insulin sensitivity

In the US Insulin Resistance Atherosclerosis Study, insulin sensitivity (assessed using the frequently sampled intravenous glucose tolerance test analysed using Bergman's minimal model, see Section 1.5.4) was inversely correlated with intimal thickness of the common carotid artery. However, this relationship was observed in Hispanics and non-Hispanic white people but not black people.

Cerebrovascular disease

Ischaemic stroke is associated with hyperinsulinaemia

Several cross-sectional studies have shown that ischaemic stroke is associated with hyperinsulinaemia or insulin resistance. In addition, two longitudinal Finnish studies (one of these being the aforementioned Helsinki policemen study) have reported an association between hyperinsulinaemia and the incidence of stroke. However, in the Helsinki study the association was mainly attributable to the impact of obesity; in the other study the statistical significance of the association with fasting hyperinsulinaemia was lost when patients with previous stroke were excluded.

2.5.1 Syndrome X

In 1988, Gerald Reaven of Stanford University brought together several strands of experimental and epidemiological evidence postulating that resistance to insulin-mediated glucose uptake and hyperinsulinaemia are involved in the aetiology and clinical course of three major related diseases: type 2 diabetes mellitus, essential hypertension and coronary artery disease. In his Banting Lecture to the American Diabetes Association, Reaven drew attention to the tendency of key metabolic abnormalities—each a risk factor for coronary artery disease—to cluster together in affected individuals. Reaven referred to the assembly as Syndrome X. The key features of the syndrome, as originally described by Reaven included:

• Decreased insulin-mediated glucose disposal.
• Glucose intolerance or diabetes mellitus.
• Hyperinsulinaemia.
• Hypertriglyceridaemia.
• Low plasma HDL-cholesterol levels.
• Essential hypertension.

Even within otherwise healthy populations, cosegregation of these abnormalities could be discerned (Table 2.3). Population-based studies, such as the Framingham Offspring Study, the San Antonio Heart Study and the Bruneck study, have provided additional support for these associations. Subgroupings of the components of Syndrome X have also been identified within these populations.

The term Syndrome X had already been appropriated to denote angina pectoris in association with reversible electrocardiographic ischaemia and angiographically normal coronary arteries (so-called microvascular angina). Subsequently, a degree of overlap between the metabolic and cardiological syndromes was reported; both syndromes are associated with hyperinsulinaemia. Additional cardiovascular risk factors have also been identified which cosegregate with the components of Reaven's syndrome. Reaven subsequently redefined Syndrome X more generally as identifying a group at risk of adverse clinical outcomes. The nature of the association between insulin resistance and coronary artery disease remains obscure. Reaven has argued that tissue insulin resistance (i.e. reduced insulin-mediated

Table 2.3 Characteristics of non-obese Italian factory workers with hyperinsulinaemia (defined as 2 SD greater the group as a whole) and normal glucose tolerance.

	Normal insulin	Hyperinsulinaemia	P
Plasma insulin (mIU/L)			
Fasting:	7	14	< 0.05
Postglucose:	35	94	< 0.05
Triglycerides (mmol/L)	1.2	1.7	< 0.05
HDL-cholesterol (mmol/L)	1.4	1.2	< 0.05
Blood pressure (mmHg)			
Systolic:	119	126	< 0.05
Diastolic:	78	85	< 0.05

An equal number of subjects ($n = 32$) of similar height and weight but with plasma insulin levels within 1 SD of the population mean served as controls. The groups were also well matched for age and body mass index. (Adapted with permission from Zavaroni, I. *et al.* 1989. *New England Journal of Medicine* **320**, 702–706.) To convert to mg/dL, divide by 0.01536 for triglycerides and by 0.02586 for HDL-cholesterol. To convert mU/L to pmol/L, multiply by 6.

glucose uptake) is the primary defect. This, in turn, leads to compensatory hyperinsulinaemia and an atherogenic risk factor profile. This hypothesis remains unproven.

Definition

There is currently
no consensus on
definition of the
insulin-resistance
syndrome

There is currently no universally agreed consensus on the definition of the insulin resistance syndrome. To complicate matters, the following abnormalities have been included as additional components since Reaven's original proposition.
- Visceral obesity.
- Small, dense low-density lipoprotein (LDL) particles.
- Postprandial hyperlipidaemia.
- Hyperuricaemia.
- Impaired fibrinolysis.
- Microalbuminuria.

Recently, it has been suggested that the syndrome of non-alcoholic steatohepatitis (Section 2.5.13) should also be included.

The following diagnostic criteria have been proposed for non-diabetic individuals:

(a) World Health Organization (1999):

At least one of either:

• Insulin resistance—glucose clamp.

• Impaired glucose regulation with fasting venous plasma ≥ 6.1 mmol/L (110 mg/dL) to 6.9 mmol/L (125 mg/dL) and 2 h < 11.1 mmol/L (200 mg/dL).

In conjunction with two or more other components:

• Hypertension ≥ 140/90 mmHg.

• Hypertriglyceridaemia ≥ 1.7 mmol/L (150 mg/dL) or low HDL-cholesterol < 1.0 (40 mg/dL).

• Waist to hip ratio > 0.90 for men, 0.85 for women and/or body mass index ≥ 30 kg/m².

• Microalbuminuria—urinary albumin excretion rate ≥ 20 mg/min or albumin/creatinine ratio > 30 mg/g.

The US National Cholesterol Education Program (2001) has embraced a broadly similar definition.

(b) European Group for the study of Insulin Resistance (1999):

• Fasting plasma insulin levels in the highest 25% for the population.

Together with two of the following:

• Fasting plasma glucose ≥ 6.1 mmol/L (110 mg/dL)

• Hypertension (blood pressure ≥ 140/90 mmHg (or treated).

• Dyslipidaemia: plasma triglycerides > 2.0 mmol/L (180 mg/dL) or HDL-cholesterol < 1.0 mmol/L (40 mg/dL).

• Central obesity: waist circumference ≥ 94 cm in men and ≥ 80 cm in women.

There are practical difficulties, however, particularly with reference ranges for plasma insulin concentrations and the determination of insulin sensitivity.

2.5.2 Obesity

Obesity is the most common pathological cause of insulin resistance

Obesity is the most common pathological condition associated with insulin resistance. There is a close relationship between obesity and type 2 diabetes. Moreover, obesity also has an important associations with coronary heart disease and stroke. Normal body fat content is:

- 10–20% for men
- 20–30% for women.

In addition to increased calorie consumption, it has been suggested that the parallel decrease in physical activity has contributed significantly to the increasing prevalence of obesity and type 2 diabetes in many populations. Decreased energy expenditure alone may be sufficient to cause obesity.

Effects of obesity on insulin sensitivity

The reduction in insulin sensitivity that accompanies insulin is almost completely reversible with weight reduction. However, the mechanisms by which excess adiposity leads to insulin resistance remain incompletely delineated. Moreover, the precise nature of the relationship between obesity and insulin resistance remains uncertain.

Glucose clamp studies

Obesity-associated hyperinsulinaemia reduces cellular expression of insulin receptors (down-regulation; see Section 1.2.3). However, a recent analysis by the EGIR of more than 1000 glucose clamp studies in non-diabetic normotensive subjects found evidence for an apparent dissociation between insulin sensitivity and hyperinsulinaemia. Thus, a proportion of obese patients appear to have hyperinsulinaemia but are not necessarily insulin resistant; how much this reflects the limitation of the investigative technique is uncertain. However, the data raise the following possibilities. First, factors other than insulin resistance may cause hyperinsulinaemia in obese subjects and, secondly, risk of type 2 diabetes (and cardiovascular disease) may depend on whether insulin resistance is actually present. The anatomical distribution of adipose tissue is an additional modulator of insulin action (see Section 2.5.3). Certain populations with a high prevalence of type 2 diabetes (e.g. Pima Indians, Mexican Americans, South Asians) appear to have a predisposition to abdominal obesity. In the aforementioned European study, measures of visceral adiposity were correlated with insulin hypersecre-

Table 2.4 Definitions of overweight and obesity (World Health Organization, 1995).

Range	Body mass index (kg/m²)	Grade
Normal	19–25	
Overweight	25–30	1
Obesity	30–40	2
Extreme obesity	40 and over	3

tion but not with insulin resistance. Glucose clamp studies have shown that lesser degrees of obesity are associated with a rightward shift in the glucose uptake dose–response curve with preservation of the maximal response to insulin; these defects are compatible with reduced receptor binding according to the Kahn model (see Section 1.4).

Molecular defects in insulin action

At the molecular level, the expression of tumour necrosis factor-α (see Section 1.6.2) is increased in the tissues of many animal models of genetic obesity. It has been suggested that this may induce increased phosphorylation of insulin-receptor substrate-1 at serine and threonine residues. In turn, this may lead to reduced insulin-receptor tyrosine kinase activity and impaired generation of the intracellular mediator of insulin action phosphatidylinositol-3 phosphate. This sequence of events could theoretically result in obesity-associated insulin resistance. The relationship between adipocytokines and insulin resistance is discussed in Section 1.6.2.

Definition of overweight and obesity

The World Health Organization (1995) defines overweight and obesity in terms of body mass index as presented in Table 2.4. Body mass index is a proxy for fatness calculated from the formula:

weight (kg) ÷ height (m)².

Optimal levels are approximately 22 kg/m² for men and 21 kg/m² for women. In men, the prevalence of cardiovascular risk factors rises as body mass index exceeds $20 \text{ kg}/\text{m}^2$. A body mass index $> 29 \text{ kg}/\text{m}^2$ carries a three-fold higher risk of coronary heart disease compared with a body mass index of $21 \text{ kg}/\text{m}^2$.

Regional adiposity

Since Vague's seminal observations in the 1940s it has been recognized that the accumulation of adipose tissue in the central (synonyms: upper body, visceral, truncal, android) is particularly closely associated with type 2 diabetes, coronary heart disease and hyperuricaemia. For type 2 diabetes the effect of central obesity is synergistic with overall obesity as assessed by body mass index. Various anthropometric and imaging techniques, each with its own limitations, have been used to determine body fat distribution in human research studies. In clinical practice, calculation of the ratio between the circumferences measured at waist to hip may be easily determined using a flexible tape measure. Measurements are performed at the point of maximal girth and around the gluteal region. Central obesity has come to be regarded as a component of the insulin-resistance syndrome. Upper limits of waist : hip ratio (which includes subcutaneous and intra-abdominal obesity) beyond which health risks become significant are:

An increased waist : hip ratio is regarded as a component of the insulin-resistance syndrome

- > 0.9 for men
- > 0.85 for women.

Low hip circumference, which denotes a decreased muscle mass, is also a risk factor for type 2 diabetes. The metabolic associations of visceral adiposity are discussed in more detail in Section 2.5.3.

Obesity and cardiovascular risk

Obesity increases the risk of cardiovascular disease

The adverse clinical effects of obesity have been demonstrated by epidemiological studies and life insurance data. Obesity increases the prevalence and degree of several cardiovascular risk factors (Table 2.5). The incidence of cardiovascular complications is increased in obese patients, the effect of visceral obesity being especially prominent. In another recent study, obesity was a powerful predictor of stroke.

Table 2.5 Cardiovascular risk factors associated with or aggravated by obesity.

Dyslipidaemia
Increased total cholesterol
Increased LDL-cholesterol
Increased plasma triglycerides
Reduced HDL-cholesterol
Hypertension
Systolic blood pressure
Diastolic blood pressure
Left ventricular hypertrophy
Uric acid metabolism
Hyperuricaemia
Gout

Causes of obesity

Both genetic and environmental factors are implicated in the development of obesity. In recent years, interest has centred on the role of leptin (see Section 1.6.2). Mutations in the genes coding the β-adrenoceptor are also considered in Section 1.6.2. Other areas of research include the following.

• *Uncoupling proteins.* These are important regulators of thermogenesis. However, mutational analysis of the coding regions have excluded these candidates as common causes of obesity.

• *Neurotransmitter regulation of energy balance.* Numerous hypothalamic neurotransmitters (e.g. serotonin, neuropeptide Y, melanocyte-stimulating hormone, dopamine, the orexins) affect appetite and thermogenesis. Some of these transmitters are being targeted in the hope of identifying new therapies for obesity (see Section 3.3).

• *Protein tyrosine phosphatase 1B.* This is a phosphatase that inhibits the active phosphorylated form of the insulin receptor (see Section 1.2.3). Studies in a knockout mouse model suggest a role for phosphatase in reducing insulin sensitivity and promoting weight gain and hypertriglyceridaemia.

The thrifty genotype hypothesis is discussed in Section 2.5.5.

Table 2.6 Risk of developing type 2 diabetes as a function of obesity in adult women. (Adapted from Colditz, G.A. *et al.* (1990) *American Journal of Epidemiology* **132**, 501–513.

Relative risk	Body mass index (kg/m²)
1	22
8	27
40	33
> 90	> 35

Obesity and risk of type 2 diabetes

Obesity is a major modifiable risk factor for type 2 diabetes

Type 2 diabetes is three times more common in the obese than in the non-obese. The risk of developing type 2 diabetes increases exponentially with increasing body mass index (Table 2.6). Individuals with a body mass index of 21 kg/m² are at lowest risk of type 2 diabetes. Compared with a body mass index of 21 kg/m² the relative risk of developing type 2 diabetes for a middle-aged woman with body mass index of 35 kg/m² or more is 100. Conversely, the observational US Nurses' Health Study also showed that weight loss of 5 kg or more reduced the risk of type 2 diabetes by 50%. Recent clinical trials have confirmed the benefits of weight reduction (in conjunction with exercise) in delaying the onset of type 2 diabetes in high risk subjects (see Section 3.1).

Measurement of abdominal circumference has been evaluated as a marker for increased risk of type 2 diabetes and cardiovascular disease. In a prospective US study of more than 50 000 men a waist circumference > 102 cm was associated with a 3.5-fold increase in the 5-year incidence of type 2 diabetes; this effect was independent of body mass index.

Reproductive system dysfunction is aggravated by obesity. Menstrual irregularity and anovulation, which are features of the polycystic ovary syndrome (see Section 2.5.12), are more common in obese women.

2.5.3 Regional adiposity

Insulin action is often reduced in the presence of obesity. Moreover, an inverse correlation has been observed in

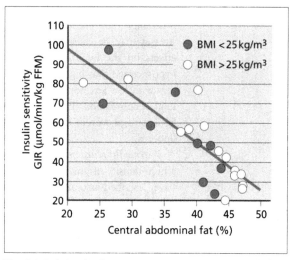

Fig. 2.6 Relationship between central abdominal fat (measured by dual X-ray absorptiometry), expressed as a percentage of abdominal tissue, and insulin sensitivity as determined by glucose infusion rate (GIR) during euglycaemic–hyperinsulinaemic clamps in subjects with a body mass index greater or less than 25 kg/m². (Redrawn with permission from Carey, D.G. *et al.* 1996. *Diabetes* **45**, 633–638.) FFM, fat free mass.

some studies between insulin sensitivity and visceral or abdominal fat deposits which is independent of body mass index (Fig. 2.6). This form of obesity is most commonly observed in men, although some women have upper-body obesity rather than the more common lower-body obesity. Case control and prospective studies have found associations between abdominal obesity and atherosclerotic cardiovacular disease. Insulin resistance, which is associated with an increased risk of type 2 diabetes, has been linked to increased metabolic activity of the adipocytes in this area. In addition, the role of excess glucocorticoid activity has been investigated.

• *Local hypercortisolism.* Visceral adipocytes selectively express the isoenzyme 11 β-hydroxysteroid dehydrogenase type 1 which is responsible for the local conversion of inactive cortisone to active cortisol. Thus, a parallel with Cushing's syndrome (which is also characterized by central adiposity) has been drawn.

• *Hypothalamic arousal.* Bjorntorp *et al.* have raised the possibility that chronic psychosocial or socioeconomic stresses may be causally related to insulin resistance via effects on the hypothalamic–pituitary–adrenal axis. It is hypothesized that high insulin and cortisol levels, in concert with low sex hormone concentrations, would favour lipid accumulation in visceral deposits via an imbalance between lipoprotein lipase activity (see Section 1.2) and lipolysis.

• *Visceral fat glucocorticoid receptors.* Visceral fat cells have a high density of glucocorticoid receptors. Recent reports have described associations between a common variant in exon 2 of the glucocorticoid receptor gene, which results in increased sensitivity or glucocorticoids, and visceral obesity insulin resistance and hypertension.

Mutations in the glucocorticoid receptor gene are associated with insulin resistance

Metabolic defects in visceral adipocytes

Visceral adipocytes have been shown to have altered responses to certain hormones when compared to adipocytes from subcutaneous depots. Thus, *in vitro* studies have shown that visceral adipocytes are relatively resistant to the anti-lipolytic action of insulin and more sensitive to the lipolytic action of catecholamines. The production of the cytokine interleukin 6 is higher in omental than subcutaneous adipocytes (see Section 1.6.2).

This combination of altered responses would serve to increase the rate of lipolysis, resulting in increased portal delivery of non-esterified fatty acids to the liver. The turnover of lipid in visceral adipose tissue is approximately twice as high as other depots. Moreover, the venous drainage of intra-abdominal fat (via the portal system) leads directly to the liver. However, as visceral adipocytes generally account for only 5–10% of total adipose tissue mass, the magnitude of the contribution of this site to whole-body insulin resistance continues to be debated. Some studies using magnetic resonance imaging to quantify fat depots in the abdominal region have not confirmed an independent effect of intraperitoneal fat. These studies, in non-diabetic and diabetic men, showed instead that truncal subcutaneous fat was a better predictor of insulin resistance.

Table 2.7 Interpretation of 75 g oral glucose tolerance test.

	Venous plasma glucose (mmol/L)	
	Fasting	120 min post glucose load
Normal	≤ 6.0	< 7.8
Impaired fasting glucose	6.1–6.9	< 7.8
Impaired glucose tolerance	6.1–6.9	7.8–11.0
Diabetes mellitus	≥ 7.0	> 11.1

In the absence of symptoms a diagnosis of diabetes must be confirmed by a second diagnostic test, i.e. fasting, random or repeat glucose tolerance test, on a separate day.

Clinical implications

Cross-sectional and longitudinal studies have demonstrated associations between visceral obesity and the following risk factors for cardiovascular disease.
- Hyperinsulinaemia.
- Glucose intolerance.
- Hypertriglyceridaemia.
- Reduced HDL-cholesterol levels.
- Small and dense LDL particles.

It is suggested that increased delivery of fatty acids to the liver from an expanded fat mass may contribute to several of the metabolic defects that characterize type 2 diabetes (see Section 2.5.5). It has also been suggested that failure to regulate plasma fatty-acid concentrations represents a crucial factor in the development of type 2 diabetes. The concept of lipotoxicity is discussed further in Section 1.6.2. Elevated circulation fatty-acid concentrations have also been implicated in the pathogenesis of hypertension (see Section 2.5.6); adipocytes contain all of the components of the renin–angiotensin system which is an important regulator of cardiovascular tone and blood pressure. This fat depot is also a site of origin of the antifibrinolytic plasminogen activator-inhibitor-1.

2.5.4 Impaired glucose tolerance

Impaired glucose tolerance is an insulin-resistant state

Impaired glucose tolerance is defined as a 2-h blood glucose concentration which is insufficient for the diagnosis of diabetes mellitus but lies above the normal level (Table 2.7). The diagnosis requires a 75-g glucose tolerance test.

Clinical implications

Impaired glucose tolerance is often a precursor of type 2 diabetes

Although a heterogeneous syndrome, impaired glucose tolerance is frequently a transition stage in the progression from normal glucose tolerance to type 2 diabetes. On the other hand, impaired glucose tolerance may be transient or reversible, e.g. by weight reduction. Moreover, even minor degrees of glucose intolerance are associated with an increased risk of atherosclerotic cardiovascular disease. As a component of the insulin-resistance syndrome, impaired glucose tolerance is frequently accompanied by other risk factors, such as hypertension and dyslipidaemia.

Impaired glucose tolerance is a component of the insulin-resistance syndrome

The discovery of impaired glucose tolerance in an individual should prompt:

• a search for other components of the insulin-resistance syndrome (see Section 2.5.1.); and
• follow-up to detect progression to type 2 diabetes. For results of the Diabetes Prevention Program, see Section 3.1.2 and 3.2.1.

Metabolic abnormalities

Glucose clamp dose–response studies have demonstrated a rightward shift in insulin-stimulated glucose disposal with preservation of maximal effects at pharmacological insulin concentrations. Abnormalities of other aspects of intermediary metabolism and of β-cell proinsulin processing have also been demonstrated. Insulin responses to glucose challenge are increased, but are insufficient to control hyperglycaemia.

Impaired fasting glucose

This new diagnostic category was introduced in the American Diabetes Association's (ADA) 1997 reclassification of diabetes. However, data from European populations suggest that impaired fasting glucose is not equivalent to impaired glucose tolerance.

Impaired fasting glucose was introduced as an intermediate diagnostic category in 1997

Impaired fasting glucose, as defined in Table 2.7, appears to identify a somewhat different phenotype to the more established category of impaired glucose tolerance, subjects with impaired fasting glucose being more likely to be

Table 2.8 Key clinical and metabolic features of type 2 diabetes.

Clinical features
Presentation usually in middle age or later life
Symptoms often mild, absent or unrecognized
High risk of macrovascular complications
Coronary heart disease is main cause of premature mortality
Tissue damage often present at diagnosis

Metabolic features
Obesity is common (present in > 75%)
Insulin resistance is the norm
Carbohydrate and lipid metabolism are affected
Relative rather than absolute insulin deficiency
Ketosis resistant
Progressive—even with antidiabetic therapy
Other features of the insulin resistance syndrome often present,
    e.g. hypertension, dyslipidaemia
Increased cardiovascular risk antedates diagnosis

middle-aged and obese. Relatively low concordance rates have been observed when the diagnostic criteria have been compared in European populations. Impaired glucose tolerance appears to be more closely associated with risk of cardiovascular mortality, possibly reflecting a closer association with insulin resistance. In the european multi-centre Diabetes Epidemiology: Collaborative Analysis of Diagnostic Criteria in Europe (DECODE) study, elevated blood glucose concentrations 2 hours after a 75g glucose challenge predicted cardiovascular mortality better than fasting hyperglycaemia.

2.5.5 Type 2 diabetes mellitus

Epidemiology

The cardinal clinical and biochemical features of type 2 diabetes are presented in Table 2.8. Type 2 diabetes accounts for > 85% of diabetes on a global basis although rates vary between populations. The prevalence increases with age; up to 20% of those aged over 80 years living in industrialized countries are diabetic. Rates of diabetes have reached epidemic proportions in some parts of the world; the increase appears to be closely associated with the development of obesity.

Global prevalence of type 2 diabetes is projected to double within the next 15 years to > 200 million cases

The lowest prevalences (< 3%) have been reported in the least-industrialized countries; by contrast, the highest prevalence rates (30–50% of adults) are observed in populations (e.g. Native Americans, Pacific Islanders, Aborigines) who have undergone radical changes from traditional to Westernized lifestyles. The Pima Indians of Arizona have the highest reported prevalence, with over 50% of adults aged 35 or older having diabetes.

Prognosis

Type 2 diabetes diagnosed in middle age is associated with a reduced life expectancy

Life-expectancy is reduced by an average of 5–10 years in patients with type 2 diabetes diagnosed in middle age. The majority of deaths (approximately 70%) are attributable to macrovascular disease, principally coronary heart disease. Patients with type 2 diabetes are also at risk of developing specific chronic microvascular complications of diabetes, i.e. retinoplasty, nephropathy and neuropathy. These are a considerable cause of morbidity and contribute to premature mortality. For example, nephropathy, as manifested by increased urinary protein excretion, is associated with an increased risk of coronary heart disease.

Cardiovascular risk in type 2 diabetes

Management of type 2 diabetes encompasses treatment of hypertension and dyslipidaemia, both of which are common associations. Drug treatment of these cardiovascular risk factors may, in turn, have implications for insulin action (see Section 3). The relationship between hyperglycaemia per se and atherosclerotic cardiovascular complications is not straightforward. Much evidence links diabetes with a two- to fivefold increased risk of coronary heart disease which is not entirely accounted for by conventional risk factors. The risks of cerebrovascular disease and peripheral vascular disease are also increased. However, macrovascular disease is not clearly related to the duration of type 2 diabetes. In contrast to the older literature, it is now apparent that cardiovascular risk is indeed related to the degree of chronic hyperglycaemia. However, the strength of the relationship is relatively weak and the increase in risk is apparent at lower levels of glucose intolerance than those associated with risk of microvascular complications. Finally, no study to date has clearly demonstrated a statistically significant reduction in risk of coronary heart disease through treatment of hyperglycaemia in isolation. This is discussed further in Sections 2.5.10 and 3.2.

Pathophysiology

A relative deficiency of endogenous insulin in the presence of impaired insulin action leads to increased hepatic glucose production and decreased insulin-mediated glucose uptake by postreceptor defect (see below) in muscle. Type 2 diabetes is regarded as a heterogeneous syndrome with the relative contributions of these defects varying between individuals and possibly between different populations.

Defective insulin secretion
Patients with type 2 diabetes secrete sufficient insulin to prevent ketosis but, by definition, are unable to regulate glucose metabolism normally. A 30–40% reduction in insulin-mediated glucose disposal leads to progressive compensatory fasting hyperinsulinaemia until fasting plasma glucose exceeds approximately 6–7 mmol/L (110–125 mg/dL); thereafter, endogenous insulin secretion progressively fails. This failure of β-cell function is regarded as the principal cause of the progressive deterioration in fasting hyperglycaemia with increasing duration of diabetes, which was amply demonstrated in the UKPDS (see Section 3.2). Failure of non-esterified fatty acids to stimulate insulin secretion has been postulated as a key defect, leading to an acceleration in endogenous glucose production and impairment of glucose disposal.

Islet β-cell mass may be reduced with deposition of islet amyloid polypeptide; this produces striking histological changes within the islets, yet its role in the initiation and progression of type 2 diabetes is disputed. Increased plasma levels of proinsulin-like molecules are indicative of β-cell dysfunction; this is an early feature, being demonstrable prior to the development of diabetes in high-risk groups (see Section 2.5.4). Transient gestational diabetes is a potent risk factor for the subsequent development of permanent type 2 diabetes (see Section 2.3.2). This may reflect

Plasma insulin concentrations are elevated with lesser degrees of fasting hyperglycaemia

the effect of increasing insulin resistance during pregnancy unmasking a predisposition to diabetes in the mother. In the infrequent and heterogeneous variant—maturity-onset diabetes of the young—some affected families have mutations of the glucokinase gene which result in impaired β-cell function and fasting hyperglycaemia. The 1997 ADA reclassification classifies monogenic syndromes separately (under the heading of type 3 diabetes).

Insulin resistance

Obesity is common (> 75%). Obesity is a prominent feature of many animal models of type 2 diabetes, such as the leptin-deficient *ob/ob* mouse (see Section 1.6.2). In established type 2 diabetes insulin-mediated suppression of hepatic glucose production (the principal determinant of fasting plasma glucose concentration) and tissue glucose uptake are impaired. Uncertainty about the relative importance of these defects may, at least in part, reflect the methodological problems discussed in Section 1.5. For example, because hepatic glucose production is inhibited at low-physiological plasma insulin concentrations, the hyperinsulinaemia usually attained in glucose clamp studies tend to favour identification of defects in glucose uptake. Glucose clamp studies are indicative of a defect in insulin action which lies at a site(s) distal to the binding of insulin to its membrane receptor. Defects in intracellular oxidation and storage of glucose as glycogen have been identified. However, it remains unclear whether insulin resistance is a primary cause of type 2 diabetes or whether a genetically determined failure of insulin secretion is unmasked. Few studies have simultaneously evaluated insulin secretion and insulin action with techniques of comparable sensitivity. Potential modulating factors merit further consideration. For example, one study of the common phenotype of type 2 diabetes found that insulin resistance was largely confined to individuals with coexisting microalbuminuria and/or hypertension (Fig. 2.7). In non-obese black US patients with type 2 diabetes, insulin-resistant and insulin-sensitive subgroups have been identified with intra-abdominal fat deposits correlating with insulin resistance only in the former. As high glucose levels lead to increased tissue uptake via mass action, it has been postulated that hyperglycaemia

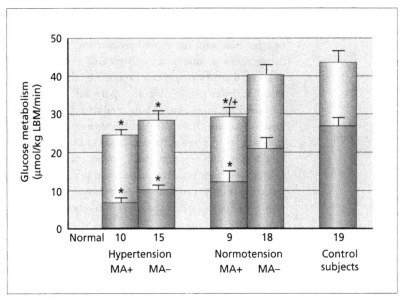

Fig. 2.7 Rates (mean ± SE) of insulin-stimulated total glucose metabolism (height of bars), glucose oxidation and non-oxidative glucose metabolism in normotensive and hypertensive patients with type 2 diabetes and either with or without microalbuminuria. (Reproduced with permission from Groop, L. *et al.* 1993. *Diabetologia* **36**, 642–647.) (open areas), glucose oxidation; (stippled areas), non-oxidative glucose metabolism; LBM, lean body mass; MA+, with microalbuminuria; MA–, without microalbuminuria. *$P < 0.001$ significantly different from control subjects; +$P < 0.05$ significantly different from patients with type 2 diabetes with normal blood pressure and normal albumin excretion rate.

may be a compensatory mechanism that ensures adequate intracellular glucose availability in patients with type 2 diabetes.

Aetiology

The high concordance rate for identical twins (which approaches 90%) is cited as evidence of either a strong genetic component (generally non-HLA linked, cf. type 1 diabetes) or, more controversially, of a shared predisposing intrauterine environment—the fetal origins hypothesis (see Section 1.6.3).

Both genetic and environmental factors are implicated in the aetiology of type 2 diabetes

A family history of type 2 diabetes is common; the lifetime risk associated with having a single parent with type 2 diabetes is approximately 40%, and 50% or more if both parents are affected. However, unravelling the genetics of type 2 diabetes has proved problematic. While studies of uncommon monogenic subtypes of non-insulin dependent diabetes have been productive, the genetics of type 2 diabetes remain obscure; a polygenic inheritance is proposed for most cases. Many candidate genes, e.g. the insulin receptor, have been excluded; increasingly attention is being directed at the regulation of the insulin gene. A relatively high prevalence of autoimmune diabetes may account for reports of HLA associations in a Finnish study. An association between a polymorphism of the glycogen synthase gene and type 2 diabetes has also been reported in Finns.

The genetics of type 2 diabetes remain obscure

Difficulties in differentiating the insulin resistance attributable to type 2 diabetes *per se* from that associated with obesity may be relevant to these difficulties.

The thrifty genotype hypothesis

In 1962, J.V. Neel proposed that certain populations, e.g. Native Americans and Aborigines, that have witnessed explosions of diabetes in the 20th century, have genetic traits which once conferred survival advantages in prehistoric hunter–gatherer times. However, these traits—which confer metabolic efficiency and storage of calories as fat —have been rendered detrimental by abundant food supplies and reduced habitual levels of physical activity. Thus, metabolic thrift has led to epidemic rates of obesity and insulin resistance and diabetes.

The prevalence of diabetes is high in migrant populations, e.g. Southern Asians in the UK have a fourfold higher rate than that of the indigenous population. Diabetes in this population is associated with insulin resistance. On the other hand, a recently reported mutation in the gene encoding hepatic nuclear factor-1α in Ontario Oji-Cree is associated with β-cell dysfunction and early onset diabetes. Thus, genetic limitations in β-cell function may predispose to type 2 diabetes in native populations with high rates of obesity and type 2 diabetes. Certainly, some ethnic groups appear to be more vulnerable to type 2 diabetes than others. For example, although a rapid transition to affluence in Singapore has been shared by all three of the main ethnic groups (Chinese, Malays and Indians) the prevalence of type 2 diabetes is far higher in the Indians than the Chinese. As discussed above, type 2 diabetes represents an enormous—and rapidly expanding—global public health problem. In the USA, the increasing incidence of type 2 diabetes in the young, predominantly in ethnic minorities, has been described as an emerging epidemic. Similar trends are evident in other industrialized nations.

Prediction and prevention

As type 2 diabetes is often subclinical for many years before it becomes clinically apparent, careful evaluation at diagnosis may reveal established micro- and macrovascular complications. Earlier identification of type 2 diabetes or its precursor, impaired glucose tolerance, would offer an opportunity to prevent or retard the development of chronic complications by therapeutic intervention. However, this theoretical possibility has not been tested in a clinical trial. It is possible to define groups at higher-than-average risk of developing type 2 diabetes. Factors which have been identified include the following.

- Affected first-degree relative—parent or sibling.
- Ethnicity—high-risk populations.
- Middle-aged to elderly (earlier in high-risk ethnic groups).
- Glucose intolerance (previously or currently).
- Obesity (especially visceral adiposity).
- Certain hypersecretory endocrinopathies.
- Treatment with diabetogenic drugs.
- Sedentary lifestyle.
- Smoking.
- History of gestational diabetes.
- Evidence of the insulin-resistance syndrome.
- Small birth weight at term (fetal origins hypothesis).

Clinical studies have suggested that the risk of progression from a high-risk group, such as impaired glucose tolerance, to type 2 diabetes may be averted (or at least postponed) by measures such as supervised physical training and dietary advice (see Section 3.1). The ADA (1997) recommends that biochemical screening for type 2 diabetes should be considered in all individuals aged 45 years or over at 3-yearly intervals. Individuals at higher risk because of the presence of some of the above factors should be more intensively monitored.

Treatment of type 2 diabetes

Non-pharmacological and pharmacological therapies are considered in detail in Section 3.

Secondary diabetes

Some secondary forms of non-insulin-dependent diabetes are noteworthy for their associations with insulin resistance.

- *Pancreatic carcinoma.* Diabetes developing *de novo* with pancreatic carcinoma appears not to be solely a consequence of insulinopenia arising from destruction of islets; insulin resistance is implicated and glucose tolerance may improve with resection of the tumour.
- *Malnutrition-related diabetes.* This encompasses rare ketosis-resistant subtypes of fibrocalculous diabetes or protein-deficient pancreatic diabetes encountered in the tropics. The syndrome has a number of other synonyms. Cyanide toxicity (derived from cassava) has been hypothesized; however, this mechanism has been challenged. Some patients may require high doses of insulin (> 200 IU daily).
- *Drug-induced diabetes.* See Section 2.8.

2.5.6 Essential hypertension

The relationship between elevated blood pressure and insulin resistance is complex and controversial. Epidemiological and experimental observations include:
- *Hypertension is common in type 2 diabetes.* Several cross-sectional and longitudinal studies have shown that hypertension is more common among patients with type 2 diabetes (up to 75%) than in the general background population. Hypertension, together with other cardiovascular risk factors, is often present at diagnosis of type 2 diabetes, the implication being that the detrimental effects of elevated blood pressure have been operative during the years before the diabetes has become clinically apparent.

Hypertension is more common in patients with type 2 diabetes

• *Essential hypertension is associated with insulin resistance.* A proportion of non-diabetic patients with essential hypertension have elevated plasma glucose and insulin concentrations following oral glucose challenge; other features of the insulin-resistance syndrome, e.g. dyslipidaemia, occur more commonly in hypertensive individuals. The use of precise measures of both blood pressure and insulin resistance (e.g. 24 h ambulatory recording and glucose clamps, respectively) increases the strength of the association. Insulin resistance has been reported in approximately 30–50% of untreated non-obese patients with hypertension, glucose clamp and insulin suppression test studies indicating a 20–40% reduction in whole-body insulin sensitivity. A high rate of erythrocyte sodium–lithium countertransport is associated with greater degree of insulin resistance. It is considered that the insulin resistance is confined to insulin-mediated glucose disposal. Treatment of hypertension generally does not improve the insulin resistance. Non-endocrine causes of secondary hypertension, e.g. renal artery stenosis, are not usually associated with hypertension. Of course, the prevalence of insulin resistance in patients with hypertension will depend on diagnostic criteria.

> Approximately 30–50% of patients with essential hypertension are insulin resistant

• *Obesity and blood pressure.* There is a well-documented relationship between obesity and blood pressure which appears to be independent of other factors, such as glucose intolerance or diabetes. The adverse impact of obesity is particularly pronounced in younger women. Increased cardiac output is implicated. Blood pressure can be reduced by weight reduction and physical exercise.

> Elevated blood pressure is strongly associated with obesity

• *Ethnic variations.* In contrast to the relationship between insulin resistance and elevated blood pressure that has been demonstrated in white and black US subjects no such relationship has been confirmed for Pima Indians. Despite high rates of obesity, insulin resistance and type 2 diabetes the Pimas are relatively protected from coronary atheroma.

• *Salt sensitivity.* This is considered in Section 2.5.9.

• *Family studies.* Family studies in white people have demonstrated that normoglycaemic offspring of hypertensive parents are insulin resistant. In addition, hypertension is more frequently encountered in non-diabetic relatives of diabetic probands.

Mechanisms

Hypotheses linking insulin resistance with hypertension in patients with type 2 diabetes include the following:

- *Insulin-stimulated renal sodium retention.* Acute hyperinsulinaemia, e.g. during a euglycaemic clamp, is associated with increased renal tubular reabsorption of sodium in a dose-dependent fashion. This is held to occur in the distal convoluted tubule which is an additional effect to the co-transport of sodium with glucose in the proximal tubule. More speculatively, suppression of plasma fatty acids by insulin could lead to increased rates of aldosterone secretion and hence sodium retention. However, the relevance of these acute effects to the chronic hyperinsulinaemia of insulin-resistant states, such as type 2 diabetes, remains uncertain. A contribution to the increased exchangeable sodium that hypertensive patients with type 2 diabetes often demonstrate has been postulated.

- *Potassium and calcium metabolism.* The effects of insulin on plasma potassium levels are well known. Insulin stimulates potassium-adenosine triphosphatase in cell membranes. There is a well-documented relationship between hypokalaemia and elevated blood pressure in non-diabetic populations. In addition, hypokalaemia may impair glucose tolerance. This is a well-recognized association of primary hyperaldosteronism (Conn's syndrome) apparently arising from impaired β-cell insulin secretion rather than insulin resistance. Stimulation of ion transport could result in increased vascular muscle cell sodium and calcium content. The latter effect could enhance contractility, thereby increasing peripheral vascular resistance.

- *Insulin-induced sympathetic activation.* The sympathetic nervous system is activated acutely by hyperinsulinaemia (even in the absence of hypoglycaemia) producing dose-dependent increases in heart rate and blood pressure. This is associated with increased firing rates of sympathetic neurones. It has been hypothesized that increased central sympathetic drive in the medulla—either primary or secondary to obesity—might lead to vasoconstriction and increased peripheral vascular resistance. By directly antagonizing the tissue actions of insulin and reducing delivery of insulin and substrates to skeletal muscle, sympathetic

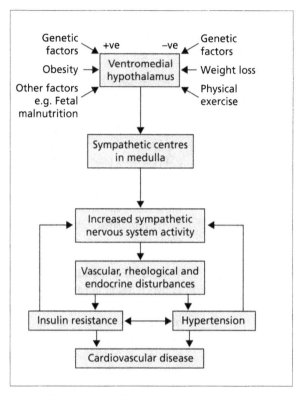

Fig. 2.8 Postulated roles for sympathetic nervous system overactivity in pathogenesis of the insulin resistance syndrome. (Adapted with permission from Krentz, A.J. & Evans, A. 1998. *Lancet* **351**, 152–153.)

overactivity might also result in insulin resistance (Fig. 2.8).

Insulin is a weak vasodilator at physiological concentrations

• *Direct vascular actions of insulin.* Insulin has vasodilator effects which are mediated by the endothelial nitric oxide system. It has been proposed that limited delivery of insulin to skeletal muscle—as a result of impaired insulin-mediated vasodilatation—could explain both hypertension and insulin resistance. However, the many methodological uncertainties surrounding this proposal have ensured that it remains controversial. Studies examining the vasodilatory actions of insulin have produced conflicting evidence of an association between insulin resistance and endothelial dysfunction (see Section 2.5.8).

- *Large vessel compliance.* The ability of insulin to reduce the stiffness of large arteries is reduced in obese subjects. This may contribute to systolic hypertension in insulin-resistant conditions.
- *Effect of fatty acids.* Insulin reduces plasma fatty-acid concentrations (see Section 1.2.5). In addition to the reciprocal relationship between fatty acids and aldosterone, fatty acids have been implicated in the pathogenesis of hypertension via enhanced vascular reactivity to pressors and activating protein kinase C.
- *Fetal origins hypothesis.* Low birth weight has been found to be an independent predictor of adult hypertension. Intrauterine alterations in vascular development or reactivity are postulated. Other features of the insulin-resistance syndrome are associated with low birth weight (see Section 1.6.3).

Hypertension is a potent and modifiable risk factor for micro- and macrovascular disease in type 2 diabetes

All of these mechanisms are speculative and the cause of hypertension in patients with type 2 diabetes, the prevalence of which is also influenced by factors such as age, obesity and ethnicity, remains uncertain. Drug treatment of hypertension has implications for insulin sensitivity; this is discussed in more detail in Section 3.5. The results of recent major clinical trials have led to increased recognition of the adverse impact of hypertension in patients with type 2 diabetes.

Reported blood pressure-lowering effects of insulin-sensitizing drugs, such as metformin and troglitazone (see Section 3.2), merit further investigation.

2.5.7 Dyslipidaemia

Considerable interest has been directed to the characteristic dyslipidaemia which frequently accompanies insulin resistance in glucose metabolism. This comprises:

- Hypertriglyceridaemia.
- Reduced HDL-cholesterol levels.
- Increased apolipoprotein B concentrations.
- Small and dense LDL-cholesterol particles.

An atherogenic plasma lipid profile is a feature of common insulin-resistant states

This interest acknowledges the increased risk of atherosclerotic cardiovascular disease, not only in patients with type 2 diabetes but also with lesser degrees of glucose intolerance or other features of the insulin-resistance syndrome. Obesity is another prominent cause of dyslipi-daemia, as is chronic renal failure. A role for mutations causing deficiency of a membrane glycoprotein, CD36 (or fatty acid translocase) in the insulin-resistance syndrome has recently been postulated. Hypertriglyceridaemia, low HDL-cholesterol levels and hypertension have been de-scribed in CD36-deficient humans. However, the nature of the reported association between these components of syndrome X and CD36 deficiency is presently unclear; glucose intolerance has also been described. Mutations causing CD36 deficiency are common among Asian and African populations. A rat homologue with defects in fatty acid and glucose metabolism (in association with hyper-tension) has been reported, somewhat surprisingly, to be protected against atherosclerosis.

Impaired suppression of adipocyte lipolysis is a key component of insulin resistance-associated dyslipidaemia

Insulin resistance in fatty-acid metabolism

Many studies have demonstrated that insulin-mediated suppression of adipocyte lipolysis is a feature of type 2 dia-betes and impaired glucose tolerance. Such studies require plasma insulin concentrations in the low-physiological range at which plasma fatty-acid levels are maximally regulated (see Sections 1.2.5 and 1.5). Other inherited dyslipidaemia conditions associated with insulin resistance include:

• Familial hypertriglyceridaemia.
• Familial combined hyperlipidaemia.

Elevated plasma fatty-acid concentrations—especially in the presence of insulin resistance—have several adverse con-sequences for circulating lipids (Fig. 2.9).

• *Very low-density lipoprotein triglyceride synthesis.* Fatty acids are the principal substrate for hepatic synthesis of triglycerides. Thus, an increased supply of fatty acids to the liver leads to increased secretion rate of large very-low-density (VLDL) lipoprotein triglycerides.

• *Impaired lipoprotein lipase activity.* Fatty acids reduce the lipolytic activity of this endothelial enzyme (see Section 1.2.5), contributing to increased plasma triglyceride levels, particularly in the postprandial period. During this period, neutral lipid transfer via cholesterol ester transfer protein enriches cardioprotective HDL_2 with triglyceride. Increased

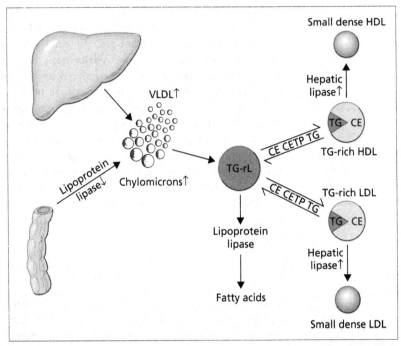

Fig. 2.9 Dyslipidaemia in type 2 diabetes. High plasma insulin, glucose and non-esterified fatty acid concentrations (the latter reflecting insulin resistance in adipocytes) are delivered to the liver where VLDL synthesis is stimulated. Large triglyceride-rich lipoproteins (TG-rL) are released. The transfer of triglyceride (TG) to LDL and HDL-1 enhanced in concert with a concomitant reciprocal transfer of cholesteryl esters (CE). All these reactions are mediated by cholesteryl ester transfer protein (CETP). Clearance of triglycerides (endogenous or exogenously derived in chylomicrons) is impaired by reduced lipoprotein lipase activity. Increased activity of hepatic lipase converts triglyceride-rich LDL and HDL to small dense particles. Fatty acids also stimulate apolipoprotein B release reducing LDL particle size. (Modified with permission from Golay, A. *et al.* 1987. *Journal of Clinical Endocrinology and Metabolism* **65**, 512–518.)

levels of endogenous VLDL compete for clearance with diet-derived chylomicrons, resulting in prolonged postprandial hypertriglyceridaemia.

• *Enhanced hepatic lipase activity.* This converts the enriched HDL$_2$ to HDL$_3$, thereby depleting levels of the former particle and producing small, dense HDL particles.

• *Increased apolipoprotein B release.* Fatty acids stimulate the synthesis and secretion of the major apoprotein of

LDL-cholesterol. This results in smaller more dense LDL particles which are more likely to form foam cells and so are regarded as highly atherogenic. Moreover, LDL particle size is the best correlate of endothelial dysfunction in patients with type 2 diabetes (see Section 2.5.8).

Effect of hyperinsulinaemia and hyperglycaemia

Concomitant hyperinsulinaemia serves to increase *de novo* hepatic triglyceride synthesis via increased expression of the fatty-acid synthase complex. This shifts the dose–response curve to the left, i.e. more triglyceride is synthesized per amount of fatty acid available. The resulting hypertriglyceridaemia competes with postprandial intestine-derived chylomicrons for lipolysis by lipoprotein lipase thereby aggravating postprandial lipaemia. The latter has been identified as an independent risk factor for coronary heart disease. Moreover, the hyperglycaemia of type 2 diabetes may also modify risk of atherogenesis via:

• Glycation of hepatic LDL-receptors resulting in a decrease in clearance of LDL-cholesterol.

• Increased diabetes-associated oxidative stress which may promote the oxidation and hence atherogenicity of small dense LDL particles. By contrast, HDL particles have antioxidant properties.

Thus, the combination of defects in the regulation of lipid and glucose metabolism in concert with the hyperinsulinaemia which characterizes type 2 diabetes provides an unfavourable and highly atherogenic plasma lipid profile. It should also be noted that the adverse impact of any specified level of LDL-cholesterol is magnified in diabetic patients.

The treatment of diabetic dyslipidaemia is considered in Section 3.4. Control of hyperglycaemia may also lead to improvements in dyslipidaemia. However, specific drug treatment is often required. In recent years attention has focused on reduction of LDL-cholesterol levels with inhibitors of hydroxy methyl glutaryl coenzyme A (statins). However, evidence is emerging which supports a role for fibric acid derivatives, particularly for the dyslipidaemia phenotype commonly associated with insulin resistance.

Elevated LDL-cholesterol levels confer a greater risk of cardiovascular disease in the presence of diabetes

2.5.8 Endothelial dysfunction

Endothelial dysfunction is an early abnormality in atherogenesis

Although clinically silent, endothelial dysfunction is one of the earliest detectable abnormalities in the development of atherosclerosis. In diabetic patients elevated circulating levels of von Willebrand factor are held to indicate early endothelial damage.

Studies in type 2 diabetes

Nitric oxide, synthesized by the endothelium from arginine, is a potent vasodilator with several antiatherogenic actions. Evidence from animal models and humans with type 2 diabetes have shown that vasodilatation mediated via endothelium-derived nitric oxide is impaired. Local hyperglycaemia impairs endothelium-mediated vasodilatation in healthy subjects.

Studies in other insulin-resistant states

Measures of endothelial function are impaired in type 2 diabetes

Studies in non-diabetic women with a history of gestational diabetes have shown that endothelium-dependent flow-mediated vasodilatation (a measure of reactive arterial distensibility) is impaired. This suggests that endothelial dysfunction may be associated with insulin resistance. Treatment with oral D-arginine reverses this abnormality in non-diabetic patients with hypercholesterol-aemia. Oxygen-derived free radicals, generation of which is increased in animal models and humans with type 2 diabetes, could inactivate nitric oxide. However, the antioxidant α-tocopherol has not been shown to improve vasodilatation consistently in patients with type 2 diabetes. Cigarette smoking and microalbuminuria (see Section 2.5.9) are also associated with impaired endothelial function. No reduction in cardiovascular events has been observed in clinical trials of anti-oxidants.

2.5.9 Microalbuminuria

In both diabetics and non-diabetics this is defined as an abnormal urinary albumin excretion of between 30 and 300 mg/day; sensitive radioimmunoassays are required to quantify proteinuria accurately, best performed on a timed overnight collection. A urinary albumin : creatinine ratio, measured in the first-voided sample of the morning, is a more practical alternative to timed collections. The following levels are diagnostic of microalbuminuria, assuming exclusion of alternative possibilities:

- 2.5 mg/mmol in adult men.
- 3.5 mg/mmol in adult women.

Clinical proteinuria

When albumin excretion exceeds 300 mg/day standard dipstick tests become positive. This marks the development of clinical nephropathy in diabetic patients. However, urinary protein excretion may be influenced by other factors which must be excluded:

- Marked hyperglycaemia (if marked).
- Intercurrent illness, especially urinary infection.
- Posture—upright posture increases protein excretion.
- Exercise—this increases urinary protein excretion.
- Congestive cardiac failure—associated with proteinuria.
- Other renal pathology, e.g. glomerulonephritis.

However, microalbuminuria is also present in 5–10% of the non-diabetic population, the prevalence increasing with age. Microalbuminuria is often accompanied by other cardiovascular risk factors. It is also more common in patients with essential hypertension or type 2 diabetes. In these groups, microalbuminuria may be regarded as a potent additional marker for risk of atherosclerosis. The World Health Organization Multinational Study of Vascular Disease in Diabetes demonstrated a clear inverse relationship between albumin excretion rate and survival. Coronary risk tables derived from the Framingham equations for non-diabetic and diabetic individuals in which the presence or absence of microalbuminuria is considered have recently been published. Annual screening for microalbuminuria is recommended in patients with diabetes because it predicts the development of nephropathy.

Essential hypertension

Cross-sectional studies have shown that hypertensive

patients with microalbuminuria are more insulin resistant and have greater degrees of left ventricular thickness (an important marker of cardiovascular risk). Salt-sensitive patients appear to be more insulin resistant with higher urinary albumin excretion rates than salt-resistant patients.

Type 1 diabetes

Patients with type 1 diabetes who have persistent micro-albuminuria are at relatively high risk of progression to clinical nephropathy. Blood pressure rises and plasma lipid profile becomes more atherogenic.

Microalbuminura in type 1 diabetes is associated with other features of the insulin-resistance syndrome

Some patients have stable long-term microalbuminuria and in others albumin excretion rates may return to normal in the absence of therapeutic intervention. In glucose clamp studies, patients with microalbuminuria have been found to be more insulin resistant than normoalbuminuric patients. Insulin resistance is not usually prominent in patients with well-controlled diabetes and is largely reversible with good metabolic control. Non-diabetic first-degree relatives of diabetic patients with microalbuminuria have been shown to have degrees of hyperinsulinaemia.

Type 2 diabetes

Two studies have suggested that patients with type 2 diabetes who also have microalbuminuria or hypertension are more insulin resistant than matched controls (Fig. 2.7). However, other studies have not confirmed this association. A higher incidence of coronary events has also been reported in patients with type 2 diabetes and microalbuminuria. Such an effect was observed in the UKPDS (see Section 3.2). Microalbuminuria may also predict the development of type 2 diabetes in certain populations.

2.5.10 Hyperuricaemia

An association between gout and diabetes has long been recognized. Moreover, elevated plasma uric acid concentrations are regarded as a risk marker for atherosclerotic cardiovascular disease. Data from the US National Health and Nutrition Survey III demonstrated that raised serum uric acid was an independent risk factor for hypertension-associated morbidity and mortality. However, the strong association between uric acid and other established risk factors for cardiovascular disease (i.e. multicolinearity) makes the role of uric acid difficult to delineate.

Hyperuricaemia is a marker for coronary heart disease risk

The β-cell toxin, alloxan, which is used to produce insulin-deficient animal models of diabetes, can be produced from uric acid *in vitro*. The putative glucose-sensing enzyme, glucokinase, is particularly susceptible to inhibition by alloxan. However, rather than insulinopenia, hyperuricaemia has been more firmly linked to insulin resistance and hyperinsulinaemia.

Metabolic studies

Hyperuricaemia is a component of the insulin-resistance syndrome

Cross-sectional studies have found that uric acid concentrations are positively associated with other components of the insulin-resistance syndrome. Significant correlations between serum uric acid concentration and more direct measures of insulin resistance have been reported.

Clinical significance

Hyperuricaemia is an independent cardiovascular risk factor in hypertensive patients

Hyperuricaemia has thus been incorporated into the expanded insulin resistance syndrome. The causes, effects and treatment of cardiovascular disease can each lead to hyperuricaemia. The clinical significance of raised uric acid levels induced by antihypertensive drugs, such as thiazide diuretics, remains uncertain. These agents should not be used in patients with a history of gout. The clinical significance of the uricosuric effect of the angiotensin II_1 receptor antagonist losartan is uncertain.

2.5.11 Impaired fibrinolysis

Thrombosis, particularly at the site of a ruptured atherosclerotic plaque, is a key event in myocardial infarction. Decreased fibrinolysis is implicated in the increased risk of acute coronary events in predisposed patients, including those with insulin resistance.

Plasminogen activator inhibitor-1

Clinical studies have revealed an association between increased plasma plasminogen activator inhibitor-1 levels and symptomatic atherosclerosis. Plasminogen activator inhibitor-1 is a circulating glycoprotein which inactivates tissue-type plasminogen activator and urokinase. Thus, the generation of plasmin, which causes degradation of fibrin, is reduced (Fig. 2.10). Plasminogen activator inhibitor-1 may also directly affect the cell migration and adhesion which occur in vascular remodelling following damage. In the blood, plasminogen activator inhibitor-1 is found in plasma and in platelets. Elevated plasma concentrations of plasminogen activator inhibitor-1 have been shown to be associated with insulin resistance in obesity, type 2 diabetes and with individual components of the insulin resistance syndrome, notably plasma triglycerides. Several, albeit not all, studies have shown a significant inverse correlation between measures of insulin sensitivity and levels of plasminogen activator inhibitor-1. Expression of plasminogen activator inhibitor-1 is reportedly high in coronary atherosclerotic plaques in patients with type 2 diabetes.

It has therefore been hypothesized that elevated levels of this inhibitor might contribute to the increased susceptibility to atherosclerotic cardiovascular disease. Plasminogen activator inhibitor-1 is also synthesized by adipose tissue. Rates of production of plasminogen activator inhibitor-1 are higher in omental than subcutaneous fat. This is consistent with observations that levels of plasminogen

Increased plasma levels of PAI-1 could contribute to the risk of insulin resistance-associated atherosclerosis

Plasma PAI-1 levels correlate with measures of insulin resistance

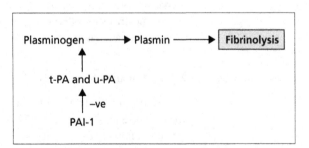

Fig. 2.10 The fibrinolytic system. PAI-1, plasminogen activator inhibitor-1; t-PA, tissue-type plasminogen activator; u-PA, urokinase.

activator inhibitor-1 correlate best with visceral adipocity (see Section 2.5.3).

Therapeutic implications

Plasma levels of plasminogen activator inhibitor-1 can be modulated by several non-pharmacological and pharmacological interventions. These include calorie restriction with weight reduction, increased levels of physical activity and metformin (see Sections 3.1 and 3.2). Other drugs, such as certain lipid-lowering agents (see Section 3.4) and antihypertensives (see Section 3.5), have also been reported to have moderate effects on plasma plasminogen activator inhibitor-1 levels. Novel inhibitors of plasma plasminogen activator inhibitor-1 are under investigation.

2.5.12 Polycystic ovary syndrome

The association between syndromes of severe insulin resistance and hyperandrogenism is discussed in Section 2.4. Much more common is the polycystic ovary syndrome which is emerging as a major metabolic disorder affecting women of reproductive age.

Epidemiology

Polycystic ovary syndrome is a common cause of insulin resistance. It is estimated that polycystic ovary syndrome (defined as hyperandrogenism with chronic anovulation) affects approximately 5–10% of premenopausal women in the USA. Non-obese and obese subtypes are recognized, the latter predominating. Recent data suggest that there may be some overlap between gestational diabetes and the polycystic ovary syndrome, women with previous gestational diabetes having a higher incidence of polycystic ovaries and hyperandrogenism.

Metabolic features

Insulin resistance and hyperinsulinaemia are prominent metabolic features. Glucose clamp studies have shown reductions in insulin-mediated glucose disposal of a

Women with polycystic ovary syndrome are at increased risk of developing type 2 diabetes

Insulin acts as a gonadotrophin in polycystic ovary syndrome.

magnitude similar to that commonly observed in patients with type 2 diabetes (see Section 2.5.5). A postreceptor decrease in adipocyte signal transduction with a reduction in GLUT-4 levels has been reported. Serine phosphorylation of the insulin receptor, leading to impaired insulin signalling, has been reported by Dunaif *et al.* Biochemical features of the insulin resistance syndrome (see Section 2.5) are common the implication being that the risk of cardiovascular disease may be increased. Retrospective studies suggest that the risk of type 2 diabetes is significantly increased in women with polycystic ovary syndrome. Hyperinsulinaemia following oral glucose challenge is closely associated with menstrual irregularity. It is hypothesized that hyperinsulinaemia stimulates ovarian androgen production, i.e. that insulin acts as a gonadotrophin. Overactivity of a key thecal cytochrome enzyme, $P450c17\alpha$, is implicated in hyperandrogenism (Fig. 2.11). Insulin appears to enhance the stimulatory actions of luteinizing hormone, plasma levels of which are often elevated in women with polycystic ovary syndrome.

Plasma levels of sex-hormone binding globulin are reduced in the presence of insulin resistance; hyperinsulinaemia inhibits the hepatic production of this carrier protein. In turn, this results in lower binding of androgens, mainly testosterone, thereby increasing target tissue exposure to the unbound (or free) hormone. Reduced levels of sex-hormone binding globulin are regarded as a biochemical marker for subclinical insulin resistance. Testosterone promotes an androgenic phenotype (with central adiposity) and has a lipolytic effect in adipocytes.

Genetics

Familial clustering is well recognized. An autosomal dominant inheritance has been proposed (with premature baldness being the male phenotype). A polymorphism in the regulatory region of CYP11a (encoding $P450c17\alpha$ cholesterol side-chain cleavage) is linked to polycystic ovary syndrome. Studies of the insulin gene have shown that class III alleles in the insulin gene variable number of tandem repeats (or INS–VNTR) in the 5′ regulatory region are associated with the syndrome.

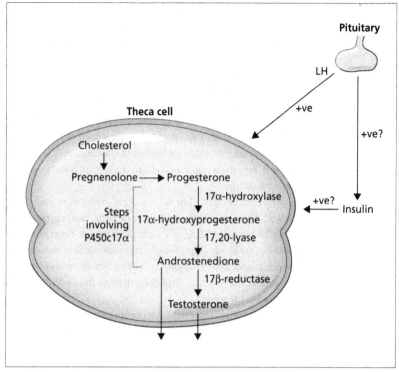

Fig. 2.11 Postulated stimulation of thecal androgen synthesis by insulin in polycystic ovary syndrome. Hyperinsulinaemia may act directly on steps catalysed by cytochrome P450c17α. Insulin may also enhance the amplitude of luteinizing hormone (LH) secretory pulses as well as acting synergistically with LH in thecal cells. (Redrawn with permission from Iuorno, M.J. & Nestler, J.E. 1999. *Diabetes, Obesity and Metabolism* 1 127–136.)

Dominant-negative mutations of PPAR-γ are associated with polycystic ovaries and insulin resistance

In 1999, a novel form of type 2 diabetes associated with mutations in the nuclear receptor peroxisome-proliferator-activated-receptor-γ (PPAR-γ) was described in two UK families. This receptor is the target for thiazolidinedione drugs (see Section 3.2.2). In females the disorder presents initially as polycystic ovary syndrome with diabetes developing during the second or third decades in the absence of marked obesity. Other features include:

- Marked insulin resistance.
- Acanthosis nigricans.
- Early onset hypertension.

Management

Non-pharmacological measures are always employed as first-line therapy for symptomatic hyperandrogenism. Anti-androgens, e.g. cyproterone acetate, spironolactone, are widely used but have limited efficacy and are often poorly tolerated. Clomiphene is used for induction of ovulation. Studies with diazoxide, an inhibitor of endogenous insulin secretion, point to reduction of hyperinsulinaemia as the main objective of treatment. This has focused attention on methods to reduce plasma insulin concentrations.

Reducing hyperinsulinaemia leads to a decrease in androgen levels in polycystic ovary syndrome

- *Weight reduction.* Through calorie restriction and increased physical activity this increases the concentrations of sex-hormone binding globulin, thereby reducing the free testosterone levels. Thus weight loss may lead to improved insulin action and an improvement in hirsutism and acne. For non-obese women, however, there is much less scope for lifestyle measures.

- *Insulin-sensitizing drugs.* Recent short-term studies have suggested a role for metformin (see Section 3.2.1) and thiazolidinediones (see Section 3.2.2) in the management of polycystic ovary disease; however, the efficacy and safety of this approach requires further evaluation. These drugs are not licenced for use in non-diabetics. Both obese and non-obese women appear to be candidates for such therapy. However, the hepatotoxicity associated with the first thiazolidinedione, troglitazone, made this agent unsuitable. Another insulin-sensitizing drug, D-*chiro*-inositol, has also been used successfully in a small number of patients (see Section 3.6).

2.5.13 Non-alcoholic steatohepatitis

Recently it has been reported that fatty infiltration and inflammation of the liver, in the absence of other recognized causes, are associated with other features of the insulin resistance syndrome. These include:
- Glucose intolerance or type 2 diabetes.
- Dyslipidaemia.
- Visceral adiposity.
- Insulin resistance.

Increased hepatic fatty acid delivery is a postulated mechanism. The steatosis, which may progress to fibrosis, appears to be partially reversible with weight loss (see Section 2.6.4). Hepatic iron deposition may be increased.

Non-alcoholic steatohepatitis is associated with other components of the insulin-resistance syndrome

Associated metabolic abnormalities also improve with weight reduction. However, transient deteriorations in liver function tests following bariatric surgery (see Section 3.1.1) have been reported; an acute increase in fatty acid mobilization has been hypothesized. Drugs that are contraindicated in active liver disease, e.g. metformin and thiazolidinediones, should be avoided (see Section 3.2). However, in *ob/ob* mouse, metformin prevents hepatic steatosis. Moreover, preliminary studies in humans have shown reductions in liver transaminases with metformin; further studies are required.

2.6 Other disorders associated with insulin resistance

2.6.1 Counter-regulatory hormone secretion

The acute secretion of hormones that antagonize the actions of insulin is probably the most common cause of acute insulin resistance in clinical medicine. Examples include the counter-regulatory hormone excess associated with acute myocardial infarction or severe sepsis (Section 1.2.1). Whether acute metabolic decompensation occurs, i.e. hyperglycaemia with or without ketosis, is determined by the endogenous insulin reserve.

Acute counter-regulatory hormone secretion may induce major metabolic decompensation

Any impairment of β-cell function may be unmasked. Thus, it is well-recognized that transient hypergly-caemia may occur in severely ill individuals with hitherto normal glucose tolerance. On retesting several weeks after the event, glucose tolerance may return to normal. Catecholamines can cause hyperglycaemia via several mechanisms:

• Direct antagonism of insulin action—in target tissues such as muscle; a post-binding defect is induced.
• Inhibition of endogenous insulin secretion—via α-adrenergic inhibition of insulin secretion by adrenaline (vide supra)
• Stimulation of lipolysis—the Randle cycle (Section 1.6.2 and Table 2.9).

Table 2.9 Acquired causes of insulin resistance.

Acute antagonism of insulin action (very common) Counter-regulatory hormone secretion, e.g. in myocardial   infarction Certain drugs (e.g. corticosteroids, β-blockers)
Chronic antagonism of insulin action (common) Hypersecretory endocrinopathies Certain drugs (e.g. protease inhibitors)
Cardiological syndromes (common) Congestive cardiac failure Established atheromatous disease Microvascular angina
Other major organ failure (relatively common) Hepatic cirrhosis Chronic renal failure

A recent US study showed a reduction in mortality in intensive care unit patients treated with intravenous insulin to control hyperglycemia. More studies are required.

Patients with diabetes

Insulin may be required temporarily in subjects with type 2 diabetes

If endogenous insulin secretion is significantly impaired, e.g. in patients with impaired glucose tolerance or type 2 diabetes, then major metabolic decompensation may ensue. Even diabetic ketoacidosis may be precipitated in patients treated with diet or oral antidiabetic agents. Keto-acidosis is associated with acute insulin resistance.

Acute myocardial infarction in diabetic patients

Glucose and insulin infusion reduces mortality in diabetic patients with acute myocardial infarction

Acute myocardial infarction exacerbates insulin resistance in diabetic patients. Intravenous infusions of glucose and insulin reduce infarct size in experimental animal models. Evidence for reduced mortality in patients with diabetes (mainly type 2 diabetes) with acute myocardial infarction has come from a multi-centre randomized trial from Sweden—the Diabetes Mellitus Insulin Glucose Infusion in Acute Myocardial Infarction study. Patients initially received a 24 h infusion to control blood glucose concentrations; this was followed by indefinite q.d.s. insulin by subcutaneous injection. Enhanced glucose uptake and oxidation by ischaemic myocardium and reduced fatty acid supply are postulated.

2.6.2 Endocrinopathies

Hypersecretory endocrinopathies

Pathological chronic hypersecretion of hormones which antagonize the actions of insulin (i.e. the counter-regulatory hormones) are frequently associated with glucose intolerance and/or diabetes mellitus. Deteriorating glycaemic control may be the presenting feature of such an endocrinopathy developing in a patient with pre-existing diabetes. Alternatively, diabetes may be precipitated in pre-disposed individuals.

The most common of these endocrinopathies is Graves' disease, an autoimmune form of thyrotoxicosis which is more prevalent in patients with type 1 diabetes. Cutaneous markers of autoimmunity, such as vitiligo or alopecia, may be present in affected patients. Other less common examples include the following.

• *Acromegaly.* Approximately 30% of patients have impaired glucose tolerance with another 30% having diabetes mellitus; insulin resistance may make control of pre-existing diabetes problematic.

• *Cushing's syndrome.* Especially with very high plasma cortisol levels secondary to ectopic corticotrophin secretion —most commonly from a small-cell bronchial carcinoma; postreceptor insulin resistance.

• *Phaeochromocytoma.* Rare; insulin resistance and inhibition of insulin secretion.

• *Glucagonoma.* Very rare; characteristic clinical and metabolic syndrome including rash—necrolytic migratory erythema; insulin resistance.

• *Somatostatinoma.* Very rare; inhibition of endogenous insulin secretion; characteristic syndrome includes cholelithiasis.

Conn's syndrome is discussed in Section 2.5.6. Prolactinomas may be associated with hyperinsulinaemia although glucose intolerance is usually unimpaired. Prolactin is one of a number of hormones with lipolytic actions. Insulin resistance has also been reported in association with hyperparathyroidism.

Hormone deficiency states

By contrast, certain endocrine disorders are associated with enhanced insulin sensitivity. Clinically, this may be associated with a decrease in insulin requirements; in non-diabetic patients a tendency to fasting hypoglycaemia is well recognized in patients with untreated hypoadrenalism:

• *Primary hypothyroidism.* Common; reduced metabolic rate and impaired insulin clearance.

• *Addison's disease.* Rare; life-long corticosteroid replacement therapy is required.

In addition, the development of hypopituitarism in an insulin-treated diabetic patient will lead to increased insulin sensitivity, thereby increasing the risk of hypoglycaemia.

• *Growth hormone deficiency.* In adults this may be associated with paradoxal insulin resistance. Visceral adiposity is the postulated mechanism (see Section 2.5.3).

2.6.3 Chronic renal failure

The kidney has an important role in glucose metabolism. It is now accepted that renal gluconeogenesis makes a significant contribution to endogenous glucose production (see Section 1.2.4).

The kidney is a source of endogenous glucose production

Chronic renal failure is associated with impairment of insulin action in skeletal muscle. The insulin resistance develops in parallel to the degree of impairment of renal function. Glucose intolerance is well recognized. Diminished renal insulin clearance may contribute to hyperinsulinaemia; the kidney is responsible for 10–20% of insulin clearance. Hypoglycaemia may result in insulin-treated patients.

Clearance of insulin is reduced in renal impairment

Decreased physical activity may contribute to the impairment of insulin action in patients with chronic renal failure. There is a negative correlation between maximal aerobic capacity (see Section 2.2.4) and insulin action. Improvements in insulin action have been reported in patients with end-stage renal failure participating in a physical training programme. Associated improvement in plasma lipids are of interest in view of the risk of accelerated atherosclerosis.

2.6.4 Hepatic cirrhosis

It has long been recognized that hepatic cirrhosis is associated with glucose intolerance and hyperinsulinaemia.
Insulin resistance has been documented both in the liver
and skeletal muscle. Hyperinsulinaemia may also result
from portosystemic shunting with reduced hepatic clearance. Skeletal muscle wasting and reduced aerobic capacity
may be relevant to the impairment of insulin action (see
also Section 2.5.13). The relationship between cirrhosis
and non-alcoholic steatohepatitis is presently uncertain. It
is difficult to predict which patients will progress to more
serious fibosis.

2.6.5 Cardiac failure

Chronic heart failure is associated with activation of the
sympathoadrenal system, defective skeletal muscle metabolism and insulin resistance. The insulin resistance correlates with the degree of heart failure but appears to be
independent of its aetiology. Peripheral and hepatic defects
in glucose metabolism have been reported. Circulating
levels of tumour necrosis factor-α (see Section 1.6.2) correlate with hyperinsulinaemia. Increased serum leptin concentrations have also been reported. Increased serum leptin
concentrations have also been reported. The metabolic
effects of drugs used in the treatment of heart failure are
discussed in Section 3.5.

2.7 Miscellaneous inherited disorders

Although insulin resistance of variable magnitude is
a reported metabolic feature of these conditions, in many
the clinical significance of impaired insulin action, if any,
remains uncertain. The incidence of diabetes (mainly with
ketosis-resistant non-insulin-dependent phenotypes) is increased in a number of inherited syndromes.

Chromosomal defects

• *Down's syndrome.* Trisomy or translocation of chromosome 21. Variable mental retardation with dementia,

characteristic facial and palmar defects, cardiac abnormalities, increased incidence of diabetes.
- *Turner's syndrome.* Karyotype 45 XO and mosaics. Short stature, neck webbing, ovarian dysgenesis, glucose intolerance and type 2 diabetes.
- *Klinefelter's syndrome.* Karyotype 47, XXY and mosaics. Features include hypogonadism, azoospermia and glucose intolerance.

Other inherited syndromes

- *Laurence–Moon–Bardet–Biedl syndrome.* Autosomal recessive; retinitis pigmentosa, polydactly, central obesity, mental retardation, diabetes and hypogonadism. Genetic loci on chromosome 11 have been described.
- *Alstrom syndrome.* Pigmentary retinal degeneration, sensorineural deafness, obesity, severe insulin resistance with acanthosis nigricans, diabetes, hyperlipidaemia and glomerulosclerosis. Defect mapped to chromosome 2p.
- *Prader–Willi syndrome.* Muscular hypotonia, mental retardation, short stature, hypogonadism, hyperphagia, morbid obesity and diabetes. Defects in long arm of chromosome 15.
- *Werner's syndrome.* One of the premature ageing syndromes. Associated with atherosclerosis, malignant neoplasms and glucose intolerance or type 2 diabetes. Rare.

Neurodegenerative disorders

- *Myotonic dystrophy.* This is an autosomal dominant multisystem disorder characterized clinically by muscle weakness, wasting and myotonia caused by expansion of a trinucleotide repeat on chromosome 19q 13.3; the predicted gene product is a serine-threonine protein kinase. Another mutation in intron 1 of the zinc finger protein 9 gene causing an untranslated CCTG expansion has been reported. Myotonic dystrophy is associated with insulin resistance with marked hyperin-sulinaemia in response to oral glucose challenge; however, overt diabetes is relatively uncommon. There is decreased affinity and defective binding of insulin to mononuclear cells. Abnormal plasma levels of soluble surface receptors suggest a role for tumour necrosis factor-α (see Section 1.6.2).

• *Friedreich's ataxia.* Autosomal recessive; repeat expansion of a triplet (from the normal of 200 to > 900) on chromosome 9q13. This encodes for the protein, frataxin, which has an important role in mitochondrial metabolism. Features include central and peripheral nervous system degeneration with cardiac defects. Both insulin resistance and impaired insulin secretion have been reported with defective monocyte insulin binding and glucose intolerance.

2.8 Drug-induced insulin resistance

Many drugs are associated with the development of glucose intolerance or with a deterioration in glycaemic control in patients with pre-existing diabetes. Some show dose-dependent effects. For example, anti-inflammatory doses of corticosteroids may necessitate use of insulin in patients hitherto controlled with oral antidiabetic agents; major metabolic decompensation, e.g. hyperosmolar precoma or coma, may ensue. Postreceptor defects are responsible; activation of the glucose–fatty acid cycle (see Section 1.6.2) may contribute. Such therapy not infrequently precipitates diabetes in middle-aged or elderly individuals with no history of glucose intolerance. A subclinical defect in insulin secretory capacity is postulated in such individuals, the diabetes being unmasked by drug-induced insulin resistance.

Diabetes may be precipitated by certain drugs in predisposed individuals

A family history of type 2 diabetes may alert the clinician to the possibility of such a predisposition. Patients with a prior history of glucose intolerance, e.g. gestational diabetes (see Section 2.3.2), are at particularly high risk.

Other notable examples include the following.

• *β-Blockers and thiazides.* Observational studies suggest that β-adrenergic blockers (especially agents without intrinsic β_2-agonist activity) and thiazide diuretics may promote the development of type 2 diabetes in predisposed individuals. The metabolic effects of antihypertensive drugs are considered in more detail in Section 3.5.

• *β-Adrenergic agonists.* Especially parenteral (used in premature labour, e.g. ritodrine) cause insulin resistance and aggravate hyperglycaemia.

• *Oral contraceptives.* Minor metabolic effects with modern low-dose oestrogen preparations and minimal with progesterone-only preparations.

• *Oestrogen replacement therapy.* The type of oestrogen or progestogen and route of delivery may influence metabolic effects. Replacement therapy with 17β-oestradiol improves insulin sensitivity and endothelial function whereas alkylated oestrogens may raise plasma insulin levels and reduce glucose tolerance. There is some evidence that transdermal oestrogens cause less impairment of insulin sensitivity and less elevation of triglycerides. Progestogens, particularly those with androgenic effects, may impair insulin sensitivity and offset advantageous effects of oestrogens on plasma lipids. Dydrogesterone appears to be neutral in this regard.

• *Cyclophilin immunosuppressants.* Immunosuppression is required for organ transplantation (e.g. renal transplantation for diabetic nephropathy). Cyclosporin is associated with insulin resistance and β-cell toxicity; similar but greater metabolic defects have been observed with the newer agent, tacrolimus. Concomitant corticosteroid therapy exacerbates these effects.

• *Protease-inhibitor-associated lipodystrophy.* A syndrome has recently been described in patients infected with human immunodeficiency virus-1 (HIV-1) who receive treatment with protease-inhibitors or nucleoside-analogue reverse transcriptase inhibitors. The cardinal features include: peripheral acquired lipoatrophy (face, limbs); central adiposity (abdomen and dorsocervical spine); hyperlipidaemia; glucose intolerance and insulin resistance. Homology (~60%) between HIV-I and the retinoic acid binding protein type 1 (that is involved in retinoic acid metabolism) has been described. Interference with activation of the retinoid X receptor: peroxime proliferator activated receptor-γ (see Section 3.2.2) has been hypothesized with programmed cell-death (apoptosis) of adipocytes; mitochondrial toxicity has also been postulated. Type 2 diabetes has been reported in a minority of cases (< 10%).

2.9 Further reading

Aitman, T.J. (2001) CD36, insulin resistance, and coronary heart disease. *Lancet* 357, 651–652.

Alberti, K.G.M.M. & Zimmet, P.Z. (1998) Definition, diagnosis and classification of diabetes mellitus and its complications. Part 1. Diagnosis and classification of diabetes mellitus. Provisional report of a WHO consultation. *Diabetic Medicine* 15, 539–553.

Amiel, S.A., Sherwin, R.S., Simonson, D.C., Luaritano, A.A. &. Tamborlane, W.V. (1986) Impaired insulin action in puberty: a contributing factor to poor glycemic control during adolescence. *New England Journal of Medicine* 315, 215–219.

Arner, P. (1998) Not all fat is alike. *Lancet* 351, 1301–1302.

Balkau, B. & Charles, M. A. on behalf of the European Group for the study of Insulin Resistance (EGIR) (1999) Comment on the provisional report from the WHO consultation. *Diabetic Medicine* 16, 442.

Baron, A.D. (1994) Hemodynamic actions of insulin. *American Journal of Physiology* 267, E187–E202.

Barroso, I., Gurnell, M., Agnostini, M. *et al.* (1999) Dominant negative mutations in human PPARγ associated with insulin resistance, diabetes mellitus and hypertension. *Nature* 402, 880–883.

Bell, P.M. (1996) Clinical significance of insulin resistance. *Diabetic Medicine* 13, 504–509.

Biaggioni, I. & Davis, S.N. (2002) Caffeine: a cause of insulin resistance? *Diabetes Care* 25, 399–400.

Björntorp, P. (1991) Metabolic implications of body fat distribution. *Diabetes Care* 14, 1132–1143.

Boden, G. (1997) Role of fatty acids in the pathogenesis of insulin resistance and NIDDM. *Diabetes* 45, 3–10.

Bonora, E., Kiechl, S., Williet, J. *et al.* (1998) Prevalence of insulin resistance in metabolic disorders. The Bruneck study. *Diabetes* 47, 1643–1649.

Brinkman, K., Smeitink, J.A., Romijn, J.A. & Reiss, P. (1999) Mitochondrial toxicity induced by nucleoside-analogue reverse-transcriptase inhibitors is a key factor in the pathogenesis of anti-retroviral-therapy-related lipodystrophy. *Lancet* 354, 1112–1114.

Buchanan, T.A. & Catalano, P.M. (1995) The pathogenesis of gestational diabetes mellitus: implications for diabetes after pregnancy. *Diabetes Reviews* 3, 584–601.

Carr, A., Samaras, K., Thorisdottir, A. *et al.* (1999) Diagnosis, prediction, and natural course of HIV-1 protease-inhibitor-associated lipodystrophy, hyperlipidaemia, and diabetes mellitus: a cohort study. *Lancet* 353, 2093–2099.

Davies, M. (1999) New diagnostic criteria for diabetes—are they doing what they should? *Lancet* 354, 610–611.

Després, J.-P., Lamarche, B., Mauriège, P. *et al.* (1996) Hyper-insulinemia as an independent risk factor for ischemic heart disease. *New England Journal of Medicine* 334, 952–957.

Dineen, S., Gerich, J. & Rizza, R. (1992) Carbohydrate metabolism in noninsulin-dependent diabetes mellitus. *New England Journal of Medicine* 327, 707–713.

Dobson, A. (1999) Is raised serum uric acid a cause of cardiovascular disease or death? *Lancet* 354, 1578.

Doehner, W., Anker, S.D. & Coats, A.J.S. (in press) Defects in insulin action in chronic heart failure. *Diabetes, Obesity and Metabolism*

Durrington, P.N. (1992) Is insulin atherogenic? *Diabetic Medicine* 9, 597–600.

Evans, T.W. (2001) Hemodynamic and metabolic therapy in critically ill patients. *New England Journal of Medicine* **345**, 1417–1418.

Expert Committee on the Diagnosis and Classification of Diabetes Mellitus (1997) Report of the Expert Committee on the diagnosis and classification of diabetes mellitus. *Diabetes Care* **20**, 1183–1197.

Ferraninni, E. (1997) Insulin resistance is central to the burden of diabetes. *Diabetes/Metabolism Reviews* **13**, 81–86.

Ferrannini, E., Haffner, S.M., Mitchell, B.D. *et al.* (1991) Hyperinsulinaemia: the key feature of a cardiovascular and metabolic syndrome. *Diabetologia* **34**, 416–422.

Ferrannini, E., Natali, A., Bell, P. *et al.* on behalf of the European Group for the Study of Insulin Resistance (EGIR) (1997) Insulin resistance and hypersecretion in obesity. *Journal of Clinical Investigations* **100**, 1166–1173.

Ferrannini, E., Vichi, S., Beck-Nielsen, H., Laasko, M., Paolisso, G. & Smith, U. on behalf of the European Group for the Study of Insulin Resistance (EGIR) (1996) Insulin action and age. *Diabetes* **45**, 947–953.

Flier, J.S. (2000) Pushing the envelope on lipodystrophy. *Nature Genetics* **24**, 103–104.

Franks, S., Gharani, N. & McCarthy, M. (1999) Genetic abnormalities in polycystic ovary syndrome. *Annals of Endocrinology* **60**, 131–133.

Franks, S., Gilling-Smith, C., Watson, H. *et al.* (1999) Insulin action in the normal and polycystic ovary. *Endocrinology and Metabolism Clinics of North America* **28**, 361–378.

Gerich, J.E. (1991) Is muscle the major site of insulin resistance in Type 2 (noninsulin-dependent) diabetes mellitus? *Diabetologia* **34**, 607–611.

Haffner, S.M. & Miettinen, H. (1997) Insulin resistance implications for type II diabetes mellitus and coronary heart disease. *American Journal of Medicine* **103**, 152–162.

Haffner, S.M., Valdez, R.A., Hazuda, H.P., Mitchell, B.D., Morales, P.A. & Stern, M.P. (1992) Prospective analysis of the insulin-resistance syndrome (Syndrome X). *Diabetes* **41**, 715–722.

Hales, C.N. & Barker, D.J. (1992) Type 2 (non-insulin dependent) diabetes mellitus: the thrifty phenotype hypothesis. *Diabetologia* **35**, 595–601.

Hattersley, A.T. (1998) Maturity-onset diabetes of the young: clinical heterogeneity explained by genetic heterogeneity. *Diabetic Medicine* **15**, 15–24.

James, O. & Day, C. (1999) Non-alcoholic steatohepatitis: another disease of affluence. *Lancet* **353**, 1634–1636.

Joffe, B.I., Panz, V.R. & Raal, F.J. (2001) From lipodystrophy syndromes to diabetes mellitus. *Lancet* **357**, 1379–81.

Juhan-Vague, I., Aless, M.C. & Vague, P. (1996) Thrombogenic and fibrinolytic factors and cardiovascular risk in non-insulin-dependent diabetes mellitus. *Annals of Internal Medicine*, **28**, 371–380.

Kahn, S.E., Andrikopoulos, S. & Verchere, C.B. (1999) Islet amyloid: a long-recognized but underappreciated pathological feature of type 2 diabetes. *Diabetes* **48**, 241–253.

King, H., Rewers, M. & WHO *ad hoc* Diabetes Reporting Group. (1993) Global estimates for prevalence of diabetes mellitus and impaired glucose tolerance in adults. *Diabetes Care* **16**, 157–177.

Krook, A. & O'Rahilly, S. (1996) Mutant insulin receptors in syndromes of insulin resistance. *Baillière's Clinical Endocrinology and Metabolism* **10**, 97–122.

Laws, A. & Reaven, G.M. (1993) Insulin resistance and risk factors for coronary heart disease. *Baillière's Clinical Endocrinology and Metabolism* **7**, 1063–1078.

Mak, R.H.K. & DeFronzo, R.A. (1992) Glucose and insulin metabolism in uremia. *Nephron* **61**, 377–382.

Malmberg, K. for the DIGAMI (Diabetes Mellitus, Insulin Glucose Infusion in Acute Myocardial Infarction) Study Group. (1997) Prospective randomised study of intensive insulin treatment on long-term survival after acute myocardial infarction in patients with diabetes mellitus. *British Medical Journal* **314**, 1512–1515.

Meigs, J.B., Nathan, D.M., Wilson, P.W.F., Cupples, L.A. & Singer, D.E. (1998) Metabolic risk factors worsen continuously across the spectrum of nondiabetic glucose tolerance. The Framingham Offspring Study. *Annals of Internal Medicine* **128**, 534–543.

Modan, M., Halin, H., Almog, S. *et al.* (1985) Hyperinsulinemia: a link between hypertension, obesity, and glucose intolerance. *Journal of Clinical Investigation* **75**, 809–817.

Moller, D.E. & Flier, J.S. (1991) Insulin resistance: mechanisms, syndromes, implications. *New England Journal of Medicine* **325**, 938–948.

Neel, J.V. (1962) Diabetes mellitus: a 'thrifty' genotype rendered detrimental by 'progress'. *American Journal of Human Genetics* **14**, 353–362.

Nelson, R.G., Bennett, P.H., Tuomilehto, J., Schersten, B. & Pettit, D.J. (1995) Preventing non-insulin dependent diabetes. *Diabetes* **44**, 483–488.

Nestler, J.E. (1992) Sex hormone-binding globulin: a marker for hyperinsulinemia and/or insulin resistance? *Journal of Clinical Endocrinological Metabolism* **76**, 273–274.

O'Rahilly, S. (ed.) (1999) *Insulin Resistance and Cardiovascular Disease*. BioScientifica, Bristol.

Pinkney, J.H., Stehouwer, C.D., Coppack, S.W. & Yudkin, J.S. (1997) Endothelial dysfunction: cause of the insulin resistance syndrome. *Diabetes* **46** (Suppl. 2), S9–S13.

Pi-Sunyer, X., LaFerrere, B., Arrone, L.J. & Bray, G.A. (1999) Obesity: a modern-day epidemic. *Journal of Clinical Endocrinology and Metabolism* **84**, 3–7.

Reaven, G.M. (1988) Role of insulin resistance in human disease. *Diabetes* 37, 1595–1607.

Reaven, G.M. & Laws, A. (1999) *Insulin Resistance: the Metabolic Syndrome X.* Humana Press, Totowa.

Reaven, G.M., Lithell, H. & Landsberg, L. (1996) Hypertension and associated metabolic abnormalities: the role of insulin resistance and the sympathoadrenal system. *New England Journal of Medicine* 344, 374–381.

Rimm, E.B., Chan, J., Stampfer, M.J., Colditz, G.A. & Willett, W.C. (1995) Prospective study of cigarette smoking, alcohol use and the risk of diabetes in men. *British Medical Journal* 310, 555–559.

Rosenbloom, A.L., Joe, J.R., Young, R.S. & Winter, W.E. (1999) Emerging epidemic of type 2 diabetes in youth. *Diabetes Care* 22, 345–354.

Ruderman, R., Chisholm, D., Pi-Sunyer, X. & Schneider, S. (1998) The metabolically obese, normal weight individual revisited. *Diabetes* 47, 699–713.

Ruige, J.B., Assendelft, W.J., Dekker, J.M., Kostense, P.J., Heine, R.J. & Boulter, L.M. (1998) Insulin and risk of cardiovascular disease: a meta-anlysis. *Circulation* 97, 996–1001.

Schade, D.S. & Duckworth, W.C. (1986) In search of subcutaneous insulin resistance syndrome. *New England Journal of Medicine* 315, 147–153.

Schneider, S.H. & Morgado, A. (1995) Effects of fitness and physical training on carbohydrate metabolism and associated risk factors in patients with diabetes. *Diabetes Reviews* 3, 378–407.

Stephenson, J.M., Kenny, S., Stevens, S.K., Fuller, J.H., Lee, E. & the WHO Multinational Study Group. (1995) Proteinuria and mortality in diabetes: the WHO Multinational Study of Vascular Disease in Diabetes. *Diabetic Medicine* 12, 149–155.

Shepherd, P.R. & Kahn, B.B. (1999) Glucose transporters and insulin action. *New England Journal of Medicine* 341, 248–257.

Stevenson, J.C. (1996) Metabolic effects of the menopause and oestrogen replacement. *Baillière's Clinical Endocrinological Metabolism* 10, 449–467.

Ward, H.J. (1998) Uric acid as an independent risk factor in the treatment of hypertension. *Lancet* 352, 670–671.

Yki-Järvinen, H. (1995) Role of insulin resistance in the pathogenesis of NIDDM. *Diabetologia* 38, 1378–1388.

Yki-Järvinen, H. & Utriainen, T. (1998) Insulin-induced vasodilatation: physiology or pharmacology? *Diabetologia* 41, 369–379.

Yudkin, J.S. & Chatuvedi, N. (1999) Developing risk stratification charts for diabetic and nondiabetic patients. *Diabetic Medicine* 16, 219–227.

Zimmet, P. & Alberti, K.G.M.M. (1996) Leptin: is it important in diabetes? *Diabetic Medicine* 13, 501–503.

3 Management of insulin resistance and associated conditions

3.1 Non-pharmacological measures

The following lifestyle recommendations are applicable both to patients with type 2 diabetes and to many individuals with the insulin resistance syndrome (Section 2.5.1). Epidemiological studies, such as the Nurses' Health Study of 85 000 women indicate that diet and lifestyle measures can have a dramatic impact of the risk of developing type 2 diabetes. Being overweight or obese is the most important risk factor but an unhealthy diet, lack of exercise, cigarette smoking and abstinence from alcohol are all associated with a significantly increased risk.

The results of two major clinical trials (the Finnish Diabetes Prevention study and the US Diabetes Prevention Program, see Section 3.1.2) have confirmed that improved diet and increased exercise can delay the progression to type 2 diabetes in high-risk individuals. However, without the frequent and intense support that clinical trials provide delaying or preventing type 2 diabetes within entire populations remains an enormous challenge.

3.1.1 Medical nutrition therapy

Weight loss of 5–10% is associated with improvements in carbohydrate and lipid metabolism

For patients with obesity-associated insulin resistance a reduction in total calorie consumption is recommended. Weight loss of 5–10% produces clinically useful improvements in glycaemia and lipids. There is some evidence suggesting that survival may be improved by weight loss, possibly independently of improvements in glycaemic control.

Health benefits of weight reduction

It has been estimated that the potential health benefits accruing from a reduction in body weight of 10 kg may amount to:
- > 20% decrease in mortality
- > 30% decrease in diabetes-related deaths
- > 40% decrease in obesity-related cancer deaths.

Benefits in cardiovascular risk factors include:
- ~50% reduction in fasting hyperglycaemia.
- ~30% reduction in triglycerides.
- ~10% reduction in total cholesterol.
- ~8% increase in HDL-cholesterol.

Reductions in plasminogen activator inhibitor-1 (see Section 2.5.11) may improve fibrinolysis. In obese women with polycystic ovary syndrome (see Section 2.5.12) weight loss reduces hyperinsulinaemia leading to decreases in plasma androgens, increases in sex-hormone binding globulin and improved fertility.

Long-term success of weight-reduction strategies

Although giving weight-reduction advice is straight-forward, long-term success rates are disappointing low. A recent meta-analysis of methods to treat obesity concluded that diet-induced weight loss is:
- Generally modest (mean 1–5 kg).
- Maximal in the initial 6–12 months of dieting.
- Regained during the subsequent few years.

Even with intensive personal dietetic support it is the minority of patients (approximately 20%) with type 2 diabetes who are able to normalize their fasting plasma glucose concentrations. In the UK Prospective Diabetes Study (UKPDS, see Section 3.2.1), weight loss during the initial intensive 3-month dietary phase averaged approximately 5 kg; this was associated with a rapid but temporary improvement in fasting plasma glucose concentration.

Thus, dietary advice remains an important initial step in the management of type 2 diabetes. Plasma glucose levels start to decline before weight loss is evident. Plasma insulin and glucagon concentrations return towards normality and insulin sensitivity improves.

Diet is an important initial step in the management of type 2 diabetes

Calorie restriction

Daily energy requirements can be calculated from the patient's height, age and physical activity. Adipose tissue contains about 7000 kcal/kg. Sustained weight loss in the obese will occur at a rate of around 0.5 kg/week with a reduction in daily calorie intake of 500 kcal (1.2 MJ).

A daily reduction of 500 kcal will reduce weight loss averaging 0.5 kg/week

More rapid weight loss will include structural protein, i.e. muscle, as well as fat; this is undesirable because resting energy expenditure—which is determined largely by fat-free mass—will decline as an adaptive response. Resting energy expenditure, which normally accounts for 60–80% of total daily calorie consumption, represents the energy requirements for essential metabolic processes, maintaining cell membrane potentials, body temperature, etc. In general, the obese have higher resting energy expenditures than the non-obese so maintenance of body weight requires a proportionately greater calorie intake. Physical exercise, in conjunction with calorie restriction, will help to preserve fat-free tissues thereby maintaining resting energy expenditure; this combination offers advantages over calorie reduction alone.

Calorie restriction can be usefully combined with a physical exercise programme

Carbohydrates (3.8 kcal/g)

For patients with type 2 diabetes, carbohydrates should comprise 50–55% of daily calorie allowance. This should be mainly in the form of complex rather than simple carbohydrates, i.e. less rapidly digested starches (amylose, amylopectin) in preference to mono- or disaccharides. The glycaemic index of different carbohydrates (the increase in plasma glucose following ingestion compared with an equivalent amount of the glucose) is also of relevance. Higher intakes of carbohydrate, in the absence of a sufficient increase in fibre, may aggravate hypertriglyceridaemia and are not generally recommended. Sucrose or fructose—the latter having a lesser effect on plasma glucose—are permitted in limited quantities (up to a maximum of 25 g/day); these sugars should replace other carbohydrates. Artificial sweetening agents, e.g. aspartame, may be used *ad libitum*. Dietary fibre has received much attention in recent years. Both cereal fibre and soluble plant fibre reportedly improve glycaemia and lipid profiles; fibre is therefore encouraged. The influence of carbohydrates with a high glycaemic index on plasma HDL-cholesterol concentrations is uncertain.

Fats (9 kcal/g)

Because of their high-energy content, fats represent a major source of excess calorie consumption, particularly in prepackaged convenience foods. Fats should be limited to less than 35% of total calorie consumption. Circulating total and LDL-cholesterol concentrations are modifiable, albeit to a relatively limited extent, principally by reducing saturated fat intake. Saturated fat consumption has also been causally linked to insulin resistance via effects on cell membrane structure and function to the regulation of gene transcription. By contrast, substitution with *cis*-mono-unsaturates may improve insulin sensitivity and lipoprotein levels.

Saturated fat intake has been linked to insulin resistance

It is recommended that saturated fats, mainly derived from meat and dairy products, should comprise less than 10% of total energy intake. Use of poly- or mono-unsaturated fatty acids (e.g. olive oil, rapeseed oil) in preference, but not in excess, is recommended. Recently, concern has been expressed that consumption of trans-unsaturated fatty acids may increase the risk of cardiovascular disease via alterations in lipoproteins. Data from the Nurses' Health Study indicates that the risk of cardiovascular disease is greater with consumption of stearic acid than other fatty acids. Pharmacological marine oil supplements (see Section 3.4.4), which carry a high calorie load, are not recommended for routine use although consumption of oily fish, rich in n-3 fatty acids is encouraged.

Protein (4 kcal/g)

This comprises the remainder of the daily caloric intake and should amount to 50–60 g/day by current recommendations, i.e. approximately 0.8 g/kg body weight.

Antioxidants and trace elements

Oxidative damage mediated by free radicals has been implicated in the promotion of atheroma. There are currently no data supporting routine pharmacological supplementation

with antioxidants in diabetes. Reports of improved endothelial function in patients with type 2 diabetes treated with
pharmacological doses of antioxidant vitamins (i.e. retinol,
vitamins A and E) have not translated into clear clinical
benefits. In the Heart Outcomes Prevention Evaluation
(HOPE) study, vitamin E (400 IU/day) did not prevent
cardiovascular events; this is consistent with the results of
several other large clinical trials. A similar negative result
was subsequently in the Heart Protection Study (see Section 3.4.3).

There is no
evidence that
antioxidant therapy
reduces insulin
resistance

None the less, some institutions recommend increased
antioxidant intake as part of an overall management strat-
egy. This approach was a component of the Steno Multiple
Risk Factor Intervention Study in high-risk patients with
type 2 diabetes. Chromium or magnesium deficiency may
be associated with glucose intolerance or insulin resistance.
However, supplementation of the diet with these trace
elements is generally not recommended unless deficiency
is confirmed. However, since many patients with type 2
diabetes have low circulating levels of some trace elements further work is needed in this area. Salt should be
restricted to a maximum of 3 g/day. Diabetic patients
often have increased exchangeable body sodium. In
patients with hypertension, particularly if difficult to control, salt intake should be reduced to less than 2.5 g/day.
The blood pressure-lowering role of dietary potassium
supplements is uncertain; special care should be used
in patients with renal impairment or in those taking
potassium-retaining medications. Hyporeninaemic hypoal-
dosteronism, a feature of diabetic nephropathy, may necessitate dietary restriction of potassium.

Surgical options

The history of bariatric surgery in the management of
more severe degrees of obesity is chequered. Ileal bypass,
although effective, has been largely abandoned because of
serious long-term side-effects. Jaw-wiring is useful only as
a temporary measure in most patients and is not recommended; subsequent regain of weight is common and
so-called 'cycling' of weight may be disadvantageous in
the long term. Vertical gastric banding, which reduces the

physical capacity of the stomach, is effective and relatively safe. However, its application mandates careful selection of patients and expertise in both anaesthetic and surgical technique. It may be considered for patients with morbid obesity (body mass index > 40 kg/m²) in whom determined attempts using other options have failed; the procedure is associated with a low, but not negligible, mortality rate. Weight loss following surgical procedures is more sustained than with diet alone. Prospective data from Sweden suggest that the progression from impaired glucose tolerance to diabetes may be substantially reduced by gastric bypass in obese subjects.

3.1.2 Physical exercise

Regular physical activity (see Section 2.2.4) is of potential benefit to many patients with insulin resistance. It should be encouraged wherever possible as an integral component of other lifestyle changes, i.e. nutritional modifications, avoidance of cigarettes (see Sections 2.2.5 and 3.1.4) and moderation of alcohol consumption (see Sections 2.2.6 and 3.1.3). Benefits of regular exercise (of sufficient intensity and duration) include:

- *Weight control.* Exercise has beneficial effects on body weight particularly when combined with calorie restriction; maintenance of fat-free mass sustains resting-energy expenditure as adiposity is reduced. Exercise also has an anorectic effect for fatty foods which may help to limit calorie intake. It is suggested that declining energy expenditure rather than increased calorie consumption may be largely responsible for the increasing global prevalence of obesity.

Declining energy expenditure is a major factor in the global obesity epidemic

- *Improved glycaemic control.* In patients with type 2 diabetes this appears to be mediated via increased glucose disposal independently of the action of insulin on phosphoinositide-3-phosphate activity. Increased translocation of GLUT-4 glucose transporters in skeletal muscle (see Section 1.2.4) improves glucose uptake after periods of exercise. Decreased hepatic glucose production has also been reported in some studies.

- *Improved cardiovascular risk factor profile*, i.e. lower plasma total cholesterol, lower triglycerides, increased HDL-

Regular physical
activity should
be encouraged
wherever possible

cholesterol, lower blood pressure and improved fibrinolysis via lower plasminogen activator inhibitor-1 levels.

• *Improved cardiovascular conditioning and functional capacity* (Vo_{2max}, see Section 2.2.4).

Exercise in the prevention of type 2 diabetes

Exercise has the capacity to ameliorate several components of the insulin-resistance syndrome. Regular exercise is associated with a reduced risk of developing type 2 diabetes in observational and intervention studies. Moreover, the decrease in risk may be greatest for those most susceptible, i.e. individuals with obesity, a positive family history of diabetes, or hypertension.

Diet and exercise, alone or in combination, reduced the proportion of individuals with impaired glucose tolerance (non-obese and overweight) progressing to type 2 diabetes in an interventional study reported from Da Qing, China. In a non-randomized study in Malmo Sweden, adherence to a diet-exercise programme for 5 years reduced the incidence of type 2 diabetes in individuals who lost weight. Important data from two randomized controlled trials have recently confirmed these findings:

The Diabetes Prevention Study trial of 522 adults with impaired glucose tolerance (mean age 55 years, body mass index 31 kg/m², 2:1 female:male) randomly assigned subjects to intervention or control groups. With individualized dietary and exercise advice subjects in the intervention group lost 4.2 kg in weight vs. 0.8 kg in the control group after 3 years. The risk of progression to type 2 diabetes was reduced by 58% in the intervention group, with a dose–response relationship between success in reaching intervention goals and reduction in risk. The risk of type 2 diabetes was virtually abolished if all lifestyle targets are achieved. The magnitude of several other cardiovascular risk factors was also reduced.

The Diabetes Prevention Program trial included 3234 patients (mean age at entry 51 years, mean body mass index 34 kg/m²) with impaired glucose tolerance (Section 2.5.4). In addition, all had fasting plasma glucose concentrations between 5.3 and 6.9 mmol/L (95–125 mg/dL). Subjects were randomized to intensive lifestyle intervention (frequent interactive sessions aimed at reducing weight by 7% and improving aerobic fitness with a target of 150 min per week of moderate activity), standard care plus metformin or standard care plus placebo (see Section 3.2.1 for results with metformin). A mean weight loss of 5% was achieved in the intensive intervention group. The combination of diet and regular exercise reduced the risk of progression to type 2 diabetes by 58% compared to the standard treatment group.

Frequency, intensity and duration

Activities which raise the pulse moderately from its resting rate to submaximal levels are necessary. The best modalities of exercise, ideally taken in combination, are:
- *Aerobic endurance activities*—walking, running, cycling, swimming, aerobics, etc.
- *Resistance training*—low-intensity, high volume, e.g. circuit training.

It is recommended that a warm-up period of 5–10 min prefaces more vigorous exercise, with a cooling-off period afterwards. Heart rates of 60–80% of maximal (calculated as 220 minus the patient's age) are suggested for periods of 20–30 min 3–4 times per week. Improvements in insulin sensitivity dissipate rapidly when exercise programmes are terminated.

Exercise has beneficial effects on multiple aspects of the metabolic (insulin resistance) syndrome

The proportion of patients with obesity or type 2 diabetes involved in regular exercise is relatively low and the drop-out rate, even for supervised exercise programmes, is high; finding an activity which the patient enjoys is therefore of considerable importance. This might be 30 min brisk walking several times per week, golf or household activities. The intensity, frequency and duration of activity are more relevant than the precise form of exercise. Strategies to enhance uptake and compliance include:
- Identifying activities which are pleasurable.
- Exercising with family or friends.
- Avoiding unrealistic exercise targets.
- Enrolment with a sports or leisure club.

The emphasis should be on aerobic exercise that minimizes any risk of physical injury. Extreme activity, such as marathon running, is metabolically undesirable and potentially hazardous.

Cautions

A number of factors may limit the exercise capacity of patients with obesity or type 2 diabetes including the following.

*   *Comorbidity*, particularly cardiovascular disease, degenerative joint disease.
*   *Diabetic complications*, such as proliferative retinopathy (avoid straining or jarring manoeuvres—risk of vitreous haemorrhage); peripheral neuropathy (risk of foot ulceration and fractures); or autonomic neuropathy (increased risk of cardiovascular event).
*   *Advanced age.* Physical incapacity, high prevalence of cardiovascular disease, effects of certain drug therapy (e.g. β-blockers).

Individuals unaccustomed to habitual physical activity have a 50-fold increase in risk of sudden death and a 100-fold increase in the risk of acute myocardial infarction if vigorous exercise is undertaken. Platelet activation and aggregation may be responsible. The evaluation of subclinical coronary heart disease in middle-aged and elderly patients with type 2 diabetes presents difficulties for the physician. The absence of typical symptoms may be unreliable and the question is therefore how rigorously an individual patient should be assessed. This will be determined to a large extent by the activity that is envisioned. Electrocardiographic stress testing is recommended for patients embarking on vigorous exercise programmes. Studies in asymptomatic patients with type 2 diabetes have revealed an appreciable prevalence of clinically significant coronary artery disease.

Subclinical coronary heart disease represents a potential danger to diabetic patients embarking on an exercise programme

A cautious start to exercise, incrementally building up to higher levels of activity, is prudent. A checklist for patients embarking on an exercise programme is presented in Table 3.1; this should be modified according to individual circumstances. Care should be taken to avoid situations which might be dangerous for insulin-treated patients, or for individuals in their charge, if hypoglycaemia should occur, e.g. sub-aqua diving, rock climbing, parachuting. Tissue damage may ensue in diabetic patients with chronic complications. The major risk in insulin-treated patients is hypoglycaemia (see Section 2.2.4).

Patients at risk of hypoglycaemia should indulge in high-risk sports with care

Table 3.1 Precautions for diabetic patients embarking on an exercise programme.

Discuss intentions in detail with your physician
Avoid unduly strenuous exercise initially
Include warm-up and cool-off periods
Monitor blood glucose levels before and after exercise
Take extra care in extreme climatic conditions
Report any symptoms such as chest pain, undue breathlessness
Use appropriate footwear
Inspect feet after running or prolonged exercise if neuropathy present
Avoid exercise during periods of poor metabolic control
Avoid exercise during intercurrent illnesses

Physiology of exercise in patients with type 2 diabetes

For diabetic patients, physiological changes (see Section 2.2.4) during exercise will be altered by the diabetic state. Patients treated with metformin, acarbose, or in some countries, thiazolidinediones (see Section 3.2.1) as monotherapy are not at risk of hypoglycaemia. However, patients receiving sulphonylureas (see Section 3.2.3) or insulin may have to reduce or omit their medication depending on the intensity and duration of the exercise. This is preferable to increasing carbohydrate intake.

3.1.3 Alcohol

Adverse effects

Alcohol may be a significant source of dietary calories in some patients

Alcohol has an impact on several aspects of diabetes (Table 3.2). Calorie load, if excessive, and risk of hypoglycaemia are the principal concerns. Alcohol provides 7 kcal/g of energy—almost twice that of carbohydrates and approaching the energy value of fats.

In diabetic patients treated with sulphonylureas or insulin the risk of hypoglycaemia is increased by the reduction in endogenous glucose production from the liver resulting from inhibition of gluconeogenesis when alcohol is metabolized. Hypoglycaemia can occur even in non-diabetics if alcohol is consumed in the absence of sufficient carbohydrate, although this tendency may be offset

Table 3.2 Potential relevance of excessive alcohol consumption to patients with type 2 diabetes.

Calorie burden
Exacerbation of obesity

Hypertension
Restriction of alcohol may improve control of hypertension

Dyslipidaemia
Avoid in hypertriglyceridaemia

Hypoglycaemia
Exacerbation of insulin or sulphonylurea-induced
    hypoglycaemia. May occur several hours after consumption
Recognition of symptoms of hypoglycaemia may be impaired

Alcoholic ketoacidosis
Uncommon. May occur in non-diabetics

Liver disease
Alcoholic steatosis, hepatitis and cirrhosis. Chronic liver disease is
    associated with insulin resistance

Pancreatitis
Risk of secondary diabetes with recurrent or chronic pancreatitis

Chlorpropamide-alcohol flush syndrome
Caused by inhibition of hepatic acetaldehyde dehydrogenase

Neuropathy
Exaceration of chronic diabetic neuropathic syndromes
Erectile dysfunction

to some extent by an acute reduction in sensitivity of non-hepatic tissues to insulin. The risk of hypoglycaemia is highest when hepatic glycogen stores are depleted. Particular caution is required by diabetic patients, especially those at high risk of hypoglycaemia. Alcohol may increase the depth and duration of iatrogenic hypoglycaemia and has been implicated in fatalities. Alcohol may be an underappreciated risk factor for severe sulphonylurea-induced hypoglycaemia.

Alcohol can increase the severity and duration of hypoglycaemia in diabetics

There may also be a risk of early reactive hypoglycaemia if mixers with a high carbohydrate content stimulate insulin release in patients with sufficient endogenous reserve. Chronic alcoholism is regarded as a contraindication to biguanide therapy (see Section 3.2.1). Alcoholic ketoacidosis is an uncommon but serious metabolic disturbance which may develop in diabetic or non-diabetic alcoholics.

Recommended daily consumption

Daily alcohol consumption should be limited to 2–3 drinks for men and 1–2 drinks for women. Recommendations to patients should include the following advice.

• Never drink and drive a motor vehicle.

• Do not substitute alcohol for regular meals or snacks.

• Avoid drinks with high sugar content, e.g. sweet wine.

• Avoid lower carbohydrate drinks—these tend to be higher in alcohol.

• Avoid drinking on an empty stomach.

• Avoid alcohol if there is hypertriglyceridaemia, symptomatic diabetic neuropathy or refractory hypertension.

Beneficial effects

Moderate alcohol consumption may protect against diabetes and coronary heart disease

Regular consumption of moderate quantities of alcohol is associated with favourable effects on cardiovascular risk factors including lower circulating insulin levels, increased HDL-cholesterol levels and reduced blood coaguability. Recent observational data from the USA suggest that diabetic patients share the benefits of moderate habitual alcohol consumption on mortality from coronary heart disease. Low to moderate chronic alcohol intake is associated with lower circulating insulin concentrations and improved insulin sensitivity. There is some evidence from epidemiological studies that the risk of developing type 2 diabetes is inversely associated with alcohol intake; moderate alcohol consumption may decrease the risk of type 2 diabetes.

3.1.4 Tobacco

In contrast to alcohol, smoking has exclusively deleterious effects and should be vigorously discouraged. Cigarette smoking has been implicated as an independent modifiable risk factor for the development of type 2 diabetes.

Table 3.3 Deleterious effects of tobacco in diabetes.

Risk factor/complication	Effect of tobacco
Systemic blood pressure	Acute elevation
Insulin sensitivity	Reduced in chronic smokers
Nephropathy	Increased risk
Retinopathy	Increased risk of development and progression

Cigarette smoking is a risk factor for type 2 diabetes

Cigarette smoking is a modifiable risk factor for cardiovascular disease and certain microvascular complications of diabetes. Other deleterious adverse effects of smoking are presented in Table 3.3.

There is evidence that, as for non-diabetics, cardiovascular risk declines with smoking cessation. Behavioural therapy or substitution of cigarettes with nicotine patches or gum are useful strategies; buproprion may be helpful. Fear of weight gain is often cited by patients. However, this is not inevitable and may be transitory. Limited success in stopping smoking points to the importance of discouraging the acquisition of the habit. The adverse cardiovascular effects of passive smoking is of particular relevance to patients with insulin resistance.

Cigarette smoking should be strongly discouraged in patients with insulin resistance

3.2 Drugs for type 2 diabetes

Drug therapy for obesity, type 2 diabetes, dyslipidaemia or hypertension is reserved for patients who fail to achieve therapeutic targets with non-pharmacological measures. Most patients with type 2 diabetes will require pharmacotherapy to control hyperglycaemia; drug therapy is also frequently required for dyslipidaemia and hypertension in these patients. Many commonly used agents have effects, either direct or indirect, on insulin sensitivity. Insulin therapy is usually regarded as a treatment of last resort but is required in a substantial proportion of patients.

Of the drugs available for the treatment of type 2 diabetes, the biguanides and thiazolidinediones are regarded as insulin sensitizers, the former acting mainly by reducing hepatic glucose production and the latter by enhancing insulin action in peripheral tissues. Other agents, e.g. sulphonylureas, may also improve insulin action; however, this is usually secondary to improvements on glucose and lipid metabolism (see Section 1.6.2). Isulin-sensitizers have recently been evaluated in patients with prediabetic conditions, e.g. impaired glucose tolerance (see Section 2.5.4), polycystic ovary syndrome (see Section 2.5.12).

3.2.1 Biguanides

Metformin (dimethylbiguanide; Fig. 3.1) has been the only biguanide available in many countries since the mid 1970s; it was introduced into the USA in 1995. To some extent the drug remains in the shadow cast by phenformin (phenyethylbiguanide) which was widely withdrawn because of an unacceptable incidence of severe, and often fatal, lactic acidosis. The metabolic actions of the biguanides are complex and remain incompletely delineated. Metformin is used either as monotherapy, in combination with sulphonylureas or thiazolidinediones—where the effect on glycaemia is greater than that observed with either class of drug alone—or, less commonly, as an adjunct to insulin.

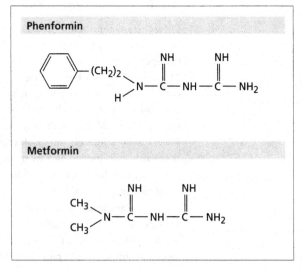

Fig. 3.1 Structure of phenformin and metformin.

Indications for metformin

Metformin reduces androgen levels and induces ovulation in women with polycystic ovary syndrome

The biguanides have been used in the treatment of type 2 diabetes since the late 1950s. Metformin is indicated primarily in insulin-resistant overweight or obese patients for whom diet and exercise prove insufficient. The drug is also frequently used as add-in therapy when sulphonylureas or thiazolidinediones fail to provide adequate glycaemic control. In some centres, metformin is continued when insulin therapy (see Section 3.2.6) is commenced. The experimental use of metformin is also extending beyond type 2 diabetes. Women with polycystic ovary syndrome—whether obese or non-obese—respond to metformin with decreased insulin and androgen levels, induction of ovulation and increased rates of conception (see Sections 2.5.12 and 3.6).

Mode of action

Plasma insulin concentrations fall during metformin therapy

In contrast to the sulphonylureas (see Section 3.2.3), metformin does not increase endogenous insulin secretion; plasma concentrations of insulin are either unchanged or decline during treatment. This occurs in concert with a reduction in hyperglycaemia; the drug is therefore regarded as having insulin-sensitizing properties.

Metformin requires insulin for its metabolic effects. By suppressing gluconeogenesis (the formation of glucose from other 3-carbon intermediates) metformin reduces hepatic glucose output, the principal determinant of fasting plasma glucose levels. In addition, improved insulin action serves to limit post-prandial plasma glucose excursions by promoting tissue glucose uptake with oxidation or storage as glycogen. These effects appear to be mainly caused by intracellular actions of the drug distal to the interaction between insulin and its membrane receptor. Direct stimulation of GLUT-4 translocation in muscle and adipose tissue does not occur at therapeutic drug concentrations. No convincing effect in reducing gastrointestinal glucose absorption has been demonstrated although body weight tends to fall on treatment; this is thought to reflect an anorectic effect. The latter property makes metformin particularly suitable for overweight or obese patients. The principal metabolic effects of metformin are summarized in Fig. 3.2.

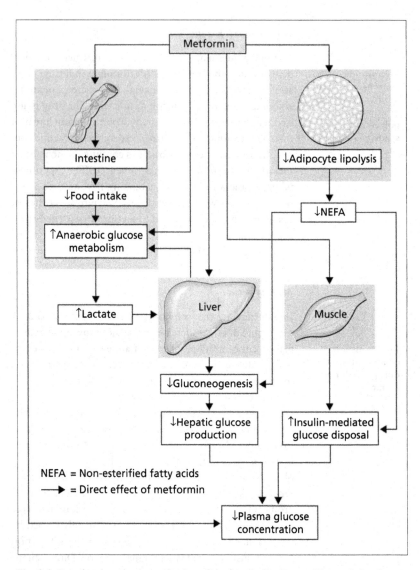

Fig. 3.2 Postulated mechanisms of action of metformin. (Redrawn with permission from Krentz, A.J. 1998. *Prescriber* 9, 67–78.) Reduced hepatic gluconeogenesis is thought to be the most important anti-hyperglycaemic action of the drug.

Table 3.4 Effects of metformin on cardiovascular risk factors.

Reduction in hyperglycaemia   Cardiovascular risk is linearly related to glycaemia
Reduction in plasma insulin concentrations   Relationship between hyperinsulinaemia and atherosclerosis
Reduction in insulin resistance   Theoretically of benefit; no confirmation in clinical studies
Reduced blood pressure   Inconsistent reports in non-diabetic and diabetic patients
Improvement in dyslipidaemia   Reduction in plasma triglyceride and total cholesterol concentrations; inconsistent reports of increased HDL-cholesterol levels
Reduced plasma plasminogen activator inhibitor-1 levels   Theoretical reduction in risk of coronary thrombosis—contributed to benefit observed in UKPDS?
Reduction in body weight   Minor reduction (with adherence to diet) in some studies

Effects on fatty acid metabolism may contribute to the improvement in glycaemia through decreased activity of the glucose–fatty acid (Randle) cycle in muscle and liver (see Section 1.6.2).

In addition to lowering glucose and insulin concentrations, metformin has variable effects on other components of the metabolic syndrome (Table 3.4). The clinical implications of these effects are generally modest and their clinical relevance remains uncertain. However, the beneficial cardiovascular effects of metformin monotherapy in overweight patients in the UKPDS was not explained entirely by improvement in glycaemia, implying effects on other risk factors, such as decreased fibrinolysis via decreased plasma concentrations of plasminogen activator inhibitor-1 (see Section 2.5.11).

Metformin has beneficial effects on several components of the metabolic syndrome

United Kingdom Prospective Diabetes Study

The UKPDS was a 20-year duration multicentre randomized trial of therapies for patients with newly diagnosed

CHAPTER 3

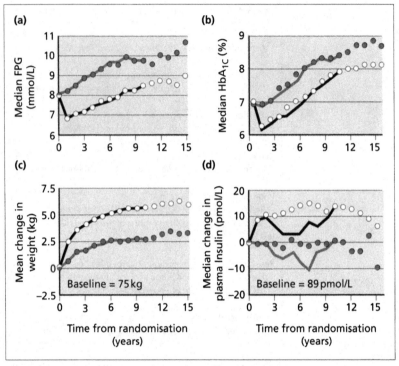

Fig. 3.3 Cross-sectional and 10-year cohort data for fasting plasma glucose (FPG), change in body weight, glycated haemoglobin (HbA$_{1c}$) and fasting insulin for patients receiving intensive (sulphonylureas or insulin) or conventional (i.e. diet) therapy. (Redrawn with permission from UKPDS 33. 1998. *Lancet* **352**, 837–853.). (interrupted lines) Patients followed for 10 years on intensive or conventional therapy; (solid lines) all patients assigned to regimen (open circles, intensive; filled circles, conventional). To convert to mg/dL, multiply by 6.

type 2 diabetes (conventional, i.e. diet vs. sulphonylureas, metformin or insulin). The study was complex with many patients crossing over between groups and therapies being added as glycaemic control deteriorated (Fig. 3.3). Metformin improved glycaemic control without inducing weight gain. Overweight patients treated with metformin monotherapy showed the following statistically significant reductions in comparison to diet alone.

- 42% reduction in diabetes-related deaths.
- 39% reduction in myocardial infarction.
- 34% reduction in all-cause mortality.
- 32% reduction in diabetes-related end-points.

The progressive deterioration in glycaemic control over the duration of the study occurred despite therapy (Fig. 3.4), including variable-dose insulin aiming for a target fasting plasma glucose of 6 mmol/L. Mathematical modelling studies suggest that declining β-cell function is the principal cause of this escape. The inability of the therapies used in the study (primarily metformin, sulphonylureas and insulin) to maintain control of glycaemia points to the need for more efficacious drugs for the treatment of type 2 diabetes.

In the UKPDS metformin monotherapy improved clinical outcomes in overweight patients

However, when metformin was added to a sulphonylurea in a subgroup of patients with inadequate glycaemic control, an unexpected increase in mortality (96%, $P = 0.039$) was observed. Further analyses have led to suggestions that this may have been a statistical aberration. The event rate in the sulphonylurea monotherapy subgroup was lower than for the entire cohort. The cardioprotective effects of metformin monotherapy contrast strikingly with the results of the much-criticised University Group Diabetes Program (UGDP) which reported a higher mortality rate with phenformin.

In the Diabetes Prevention Program metformin (in concert with lifestyle advice) reduced the risk of progression from impaired glucose tolerance to type 2 diabetes by 31% over 3 years (see Section 3.1.2).

Pharmacokinetics

Metformin is absorbed predominantly from the small intestine, attaining high local concentrations. The bioavailability of an oral dose is 50–60%; the mean plasma half-life is between 2 and 3 h, necessitating 2–3 daily doses. Metformin is not bound to plasma proteins (cf. 12–20% binding for phenformin) and is therefore not subject to displacement by other drugs. No hepatic metabolism occurs, virtually all of the drug being excreted unchanged in the urine; the drug is secreted by renal tubules.

Adverse effects

Gastrointestinal symptoms
These are encountered in 5–20% of patients. Symptoms include nausea, anorexia, abdominal discomfort and

**Gastrointestinal
side-effects of
metformin prove
intolerable for
many patients**

diarrhoea; symptoms resolve rapidly on withdrawal. A few
patients are unable to tolerate these effects and compliance
may be reduced in other patients.

Dose-titration, introducing metformin at a low dose—
500 mg/day for the first week—can help reduce the frequency and severity of gastrointestinal symptoms which
may prove to be transient. The dose is subsequently increased to 500 mg t.d.s or 850 mg b.d. A dose–response
effect is evident up to 3 g daily.

Other side-effects are rare. Although reduced serum concentrations of vitamin B_{12} and folate are well documented,
clinical deficiencies are exceptionally uncommon.

Lactate metabolism

**Lactic acidosis is a
rare but potentially
lethal complication
of biguanide
therapy**

Lactate metabolism has been the primary safety concern
because of the association between these drugs and lactic
acidosis. For metformin, the risk of fatality from lactic acidosis is estimated to be similar to that from sulphonylurea-
induced hypoglycaemia. Unlike phenformin, which binds
to mitochondrial membranes with high affinity thereby
inhibiting lactate oxidation, metformin has only minor
effects on blood lactate unless concentrations of the drug
rise to toxic levels. The intrinsic risk of lactic acidosis is considerably lower with metformin than phenformin and most
reported cases of metformin-associated lactic acidosis have
been encountered in patients with contraindications to its
use (Table 3.5).

**Contraindications
to metformin
should be carefully
observed**

There is controversy in the literature concerning the relevance of metformin accumulation to lactic acidosis. None
the less, although rare, lactic acidosis in metformin-treated
patients carries a high case-fatality rate. When the drug was
introduced into the USA in 1995 the contraindications to
its use were reaffirmed; many clinicians pursue a cautious
approach which may have contributed to the low rate of
reported lactic acidosis in the UK and elsewhere. However,
there is evidence from hospital-based and population studies
that many patients with contraindications receive metformin inappropriately.

The principal contraindication is renal impairment because
this leads to accumulation of metformin. Care should
therefore be exercised even in patients with proteinuria,
the earliest clinical indicator of diabetic nephropathy; renal

Table 3.5 Principal contraindications to metformin.

Contraindication	Comments
Renal impairment	Withdraw metformin if plasma creatinine is elevated; risk of drug accumulation
Cardiac failure	Avoid use in cardiac decompensation; increased lactate production and reduced hepatic lactate clearance
Ischaemic heart disease	Avoid in patients with recent myocardial infarction; withdraw and use intravenous insulin-dextrose infusion during acute myocardial infarction
Alcoholism	Avoid; hyperlactataemia
Hepatic impairment	Avoid; hyperlactatamaemia secondary to reduced lactate clearance
Severe sepsis	Withdraw; risk of hyperlactataemia
Surgery	Avoid perioperatively; use insulin if necessary
Peripheral vascular disease	Avoid; increased lactate generation
Chronic pulmonary disease	Avoid; risk of hypoxia and hyperlactaemia
Radiological contrast studies	Withdraw temporarily; maintain adequate hydration

function should be checked annually. Metformin should also be avoided in clinical conditions in which:

• Lactate production is increased (e.g. cardiopulmonary decompensation or peripheral vascular disease).
• Hepatic clearance is impaired (e.g. alcoholism).

Renal impairment is the principal contraindication to metformin therapy

In common with all prescribing, the risks and benefits of therapy must be carefully considered for each patient.

Hypoglycaemia

A noteworthy aspect of metformin is the virtual absence of risk of hypoglycaemia when used as monotherapy, even when taken in overdose. This protection may be a consequence of continued delivery of lactate (derived from the splanchnic bed) and other gluconeogenic precursors which help to sustain hepatic glucose production as plasma glucose levels decline. However, metformin may potentiate the hypoglycaemic effects of sulphonylureas and insulin.

139

Drug interactions

The renal clearance of metformin is reduced by cimetidine and a dosage reduction may be appropriate in these circumstances.

3.2.2 Thiazolidinediones

The thiazolidinediones enhance or mimic the actions of insulin

The thiazolidinediones are a recently introduced class of drugs that have the effect of enhancing certain metabolic actions of insulin. These agents represent a major advance in the treatment of type 2 diabetes.

The first to reach the market was troglitazone (see Fig. 3.4). However, the drug was withdrawn by its UK distributors shortly after launch in 1997 following reports from the

Troglitazone, the first drug in the class, was withdrawn in the UK shortly after its introduction

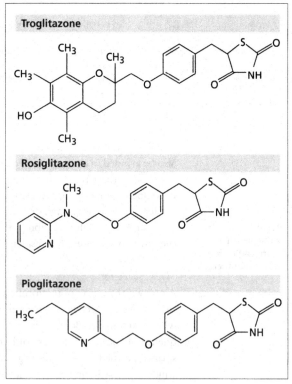

Fig. 3.4 Structures of troglitazone, rosiglitazone and pioglitazone.

Troglitazone was withdrawn in in the USA and elsewhere in 2000

USA of severe hepatotoxicity, including fatalities. Troglitazone was withdrawn in the USA and elsewhere in March 2000. This followed amendments to the product licence that in-cluded increased frequency of monitoring of liver function tests and curtailment of use as monotherapy. Troglitazone continues to be available in some countries. The more potent agents, rosiglitazone and piogli-tazone (see Fig. 3.4), were introduced in the USA in 1999. The issue of hepatoxicity is discussed in more detail below.

Clinical indications for the thiazolidinediones

Rosiglitazone and pioglitazone were introduced in Europe in 2000

Rosiglitazone was launched in Europe in July 2000 with pioglitazone following later in the same year. In contrast to the USA, the drugs are not approved as monotherapy or combination with insulin (pioglitazone is licenced for the latter in the USA). Rosiglitazone and pioglitazone may be used in Europe when glycaemic control is inadequate despite maximally tolerated doses of metformin or sulphonylureas:
• In combination with a sulphonylurea if metformin is contraindicated or not tolerated.
• In obese patients in combination with metformin.

Mode of action

Both rosiglitazone and pioglitazone have been evaluated by the UK National Institute for Clinical Excellence (NICE)

Thiazolidinediones have effects on both lipid and glucose metabolism:
• Increased fatty acid uptake by adipose tissue.
• Improved glucose disposal in peripheral tissues.
Effects on hepatic glucose production are less clear. These actions are thought to be mediated via effects of the drugs with a specific nuclear receptor, the peroxisome proliferator-activated-receptor-gamma (PPAR-γ); direct effects on intra-cellular glucose transporters have also been reported. PPAR-γ is a member of the superfamily of nuclear receptors that is predominantly expressed in adipocytes; lesser ex-pression occurs in tissues such as skeletal muscle and liver. Mutations of PPAR-γ have recently been described

Activation of nuclear PPAR-γ receptors is a major action of thiazolidinediones

that result in insulin resistance (see Section 2.5.12). Other polymorphisms (e.g. the Pro12→Ala mutation in the PPAR-γ2-specific exon B) are associated with improved insulin sensitivity and lower body mass index. Activation

141

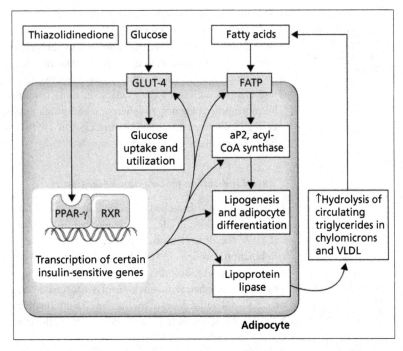

Fig. 3.5 Thiazolidinediones (TZD) bind to the complex of the peroxisome proliferator-activated receptor-γ and retinoid X receptor (PPAR-γ-RXR) causing transcription of insulin-sensitive genes involved in glucose uptake and lipogenesis. Abbreviations: FATP = fatty acid transporter protein; GLUT-4 = glucose transporter isoform 4; aP2 = adipocyte fatty-acid binding protein; VLDL = very low density lipoproteins. Reproduced with permission from Krentz, A.J. & Bailey, C.J. 2001. Type 2 diabetes in practice, p. 148.

of PPAR-γ increases transcription of insulin-sensitive genes influencing adipocyte differentiation and function (Fig. 3.5). The active form of PPAR-γ is a heterodimer with the retinoid-X receptor. The complex then binds to response elements in nuclear DNA.

Binding of thiazolidinediones ultimately alters the expression of insulin-sensitive genes involved in the regulation of lipid and carbohydrate metabolism including:

- Lipoprotein lipase.
- Fatty acid transporter protein.
- Fatty acyl CoA-synthase.
- Malic enzyme.
- Glucokinase.

The combined effect is to increase the uptake of circulating non-esterified fatty acids and increase lipogenesis within adipocytes. The precise mechanisms through which these drugs improve insulin sensitivity in glucose metabolism remains to be determined. In animal models, expression and translocation of GLUT-4 facilitative glucose transporters occurs in adipocytes; the inhibitory effect of tumour necrosis factor-γ (Section 1.6.2) on insulin-stimulated glucose uptake is also blocked by thiazolidinediones. Levels of resistin and leptin are also reduced (see Section 1.6.2). Thiazolidinediones have an affinity for PPAR-γ in the nanomolar range, in contrast to putative naturally occurring ligands such as fatty acids which have to be present in much higher concentrations. PPAR receptors are also expressed in all vascular cell types where they exert anti-inflammatory actions.

Thiazolidinediones require insulin to exert effects on glucose metabolism

As with biguanides, thiazolidinediones require the presence of insulin in order to exert effects on glucose metabolism. The maximal glucose-lowering effects of thiazolidines takes approximately 6–8 weeks to become fully apparent.

Glucose-lowering effects are maximal after 6–8 weeks' of therapy

No thiazolidinediones are currently licensed for use as monotherapy in Europe

Efficacy as monotherapy

As monotherapy (200 mg to 600 mg daily), troglitazone produced a dose-dependent lowering of blood glucose levels of a magnitude similar to either a sulphonylurea or metformin (i.e. by approximately 15–25%). Combining troglitazone (or other thiazolidinediones) with sulphonylureas or metformin enhanced the glucose-lowering effect. Combining troglitazone or pioglitazone (in the USA) with exogenous insulin allowed insulin doses to be reduced substantially in obese patients, with a concomitant improvement in glycaemic control. In addition to its glucose-lowering action troglitazone and other drugs in this class cause dose-dependent reductions in fasting plasma concentrations of:

- Insulin.
- C-peptide.
- Non-esterified fatty acids.
- Triglycerides (troglitazone and pioglitazone).

Enhanced insulin action in glucose metabolism has been confirmed using the glucose clamp technique with

Increases in
LDL-cholesterol
and HDL-
cholesterol have
been reported with
troglitazone

improvements of up to 50% in insulin-mediated glucose disposal. Predictably, obese insulin resistant patients appear to be more likely to respond. The overall decline in HbA_{1c} with troglitazone observed in trials was approximately 1.0%. Effects on other aspects of lipid metabolism included a rise in cardioprotective HDL-cholesterol; however, LDL-cholesterol also increased, although apoplipoprotein B levels were unchanged. The effects on fatty acids and triglycerides appeared to be less dependent on the presence of circulating insulin than the effect on blood glucose.

Rosiglitazone and pioglitazone also have effects on circulating lipids. However, pioglitazone appears to have less pronounced effects on LDL-cholesterol allied to reductions in triglycerides. The relevance of the anti-oxidant effects of troglitazone (which uniquely contains a vitamin E moiety; see Fig. 3.4) remain uncertain. Rosiglitazone lowers blood pressure and protects against endothelial dysfunction in the insulin-resistant Zucker fatty rat. On a molar basis, rosiglitazone is more potent than troglitazone or pioglitazone; 4–8 mg daily of rosiglitazone appears to be comparable to 200–800 mg troglitazone or 30–45 mg pioglitazone in terms of glucose-lowering effect. This reflects higher binding affinity of rosiglitazone for intact adipocytes expressing PPAR-γ. Both rosiglitazone and pioglitazone appear to be more effective at reducing HbA_{1c} levels as monotherapy than troglitazone (approximately –1.5% and –1.8%, respectively). The efficacy of rosiglitazone was assessed in a 12 week placebo-controlled dose-ranging trial involving 380 patients with type 2 diabetes (311 of whom completed the study). Other oral agents were withdrawn for 4–7 weeks before randomization to rosiglitazone (0.05 mg to 1.0 mg b.d.) or placebo. Rosiglitazone produced significant decreases in fasting plasma glucose (Fig. 3.6) and fructosamine at doses of 1.0 and 2.0 mg b.d.

At 2.0 mg b.d. significant decrements in plasma insulin and fatty acids were observed. Patients with a body mass index >27 kg/m² had greater decreases in fasting glucose levels than less overweight patients (–2.2. vs. –1.1 mmol/L, respectively). Plasma total, LDL and HDL cholesterol concentrations increased significantly at 2.0 mg b.d. However, neither triglycerides nor the total/HDL cholesterol ratio altered significantly. Weight gain correlated with improve-

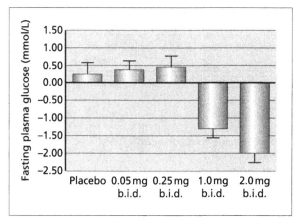

Fig. 3.6 Mean changes from baseline in fasting plasma glucose after 12 weeks of treatment with rosiglitazone (intention-to-treat population). Data are mean ± SE. (Reproduced with permission from Patel, J. *et al.* 1999. *Diabetes, Obesity & Metabolism* 1, 165–172.)

ment in glycaemic control and was considered to be clinically insignificant (maximum mean weight gain 0.36 kg at the highest dose). In this study, rosiglitazone had an adverse event frequency comparable to placebo. One patient treated with 1.0 mg b.d. had a transient elevation of alanine aminotransferase to >3.0 the upper limit of the reference range which decreased with continued treatment. No clinically significant changes were observed in haematocrit, left ventricular mass (as determined by echocardiography) or blood pressure.

Combination therapy

Troglitazone, rosiglitazone and pioglitazone have also been evaluated in combination with sulphonylureas or metformin. In general, glucose-lowering effects are more marked in combination with a sulphonylurea, less potent when combined with metformin and lowest as monotherapy. No clear difference has emerged in glucose-lowering effects between rosiglitazone and pioglitazone (Table 3.6) In a 16 week study, troglitazone 100 mg or 200 mg daily was added to sulphonylurea-treated patients producing significant improvements in glycaemic control at both doses. The reduction from baseline in fasting blood glucose at the

Table 3.6 Blood glucose-lowering effects of rosiglitazone and pioglitazone in type 2 diabetic patients. Data from published abstracts.

	Dose (mg/day)	Duration (weeks)	↓ FPG* (mmol/L)	↓ HbA$_{1E}$* (%)
Monotherapy				
Rosiglitazone	8	26	3.0	0.6
Pioglitazone	30	16	2.8	0.6
Combination with sulphonylurea[†]				
Rosiglitazone	4	26	2.1	0.9
Pioglitazone	30	16	2.9	1.2
Combination with metformin[†]				
Rosiglitazone	8	26	2.7	0.8
Pioglitazone	30	16	2.4	0.6
Combination with insulin				
Rosiglitazone	8	26	2.5	1.2[a]
Pioglitazone	30	16	2.7	1.2[b]

Abbreviations: FPG = fasting plasma glucose; * = decrease from baseline; † = patients poorly controlled on existing treatment before rosiglitazone or pioglitazone added in; a = average decrease in insulin dose of 9 units/day; b = 16% of patients reduced their insulin dose by > 25%. Reproduced with permission from Krentz, A.J. & Bailey, C.J. 2001. *Type 2 Diabetes in Practice*, p. 150, Royal Society of Medicine Press, London.

higher dose was approximately 1.0 mmol/L; fasting glucose rose non-significantly in the sulphonylurea monotherapy group. Compared with metformin, troglitazone more effectively stimulated glucose disposal, whereas the former drug produced a greater suppression of hepatic glucose production (Fig. 3.7). When troglitazone was added to metformin, a significant further decrease in insulin-mediated glucose disposal was accompanied by a reduction in glycated haemoglobin.

In a US multicentre trial, pioglitazone (30 mg daily) added to metformin improved both glycaemic control and plasma lipids (with a decrease in triglycerides, an increase in HDL-cholesterol and a decrease in total cholesterol/HDL-cholesterol ratio). In a 16 week study involving 560 patients addition of pioglitazone to sulphonylurea therapy significantly improved glycaemic control (Fig. 3.8). Fasting plasma glucose also showed a dose-dependent reduction of

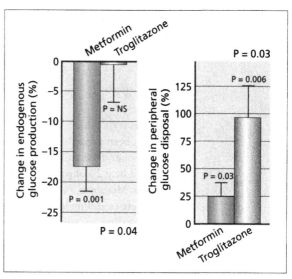

Fig. 3.7 Mean (± SE) changes in hepatic glucose production and glucose disposal in patients with type 2 diabetes who received either metformin or troglitazone for 3 months. (Reproduced with permission from Inzucchi, S.E. *et al.* 1998. *New England Journal of Medicine* **338**, 867–872.)

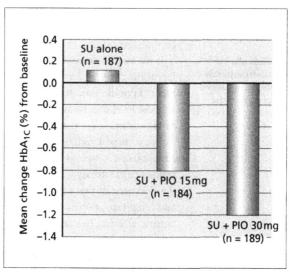

Fig 3.8 Effect of addition of pioglitazone 15 mg or 30 mg daily on HbA$_{1c}$ levels in 560 sulphonylurea-treated patients. Data with permission from Schneider, R. *et al.* (1999) *Diabetes* **48** (suppl. 1), 106.

1.9 mmol/L (15 mg) and 2.9 mmol/L (30 mg). Plasma lipid profiles also improved with an increase in HDL-cholesterol and a reduction in triglycerides.

Adverse effects

Hepatoxicity

This has been proved ultimately to be a major issue with troglitazone. Discontinuation of the drug occurred in approximately 2% of patients because of elevations of liver enzymes. Moreover, by March 2000, 90 cases of fulminant liver failure (resulting in the deaths of 63 patients and liver transplantation in some others) had been linked with exposure to the drug. The drug was withdrawn from the Diabetes Prevention Program for this reason (see Section 3.1.2). Hepatotoxicity was mainly been encountered during the first six months of therapy and was usually reversible on discontinuation of the drug. This devastating side-effect became apparent only in phase IV, i.e. post-marketing. Thiazolidinediones are presently contraindicated in patients with elevations of plasma alanine aminotranserase >2.5 of the upper limit of the reference range. Clinical evidence of liver disease serves as another contraindication.

Thiazolidinediones are contraindicated in patients with liver disease

It has been recommended that alanine aminotransferase be measured every 2 months during the first year of treatment. Periodic monitoring is advised thereafter. If transaminase level rises to more than three times the upper limit of the normal range therapy should be discontinued.

Plasma alanine aminotransferase must be measured every 2 months during the first year of therapy

In excess of 1 million patients have now received either rosiglitazone or pioglitazone with no clear evidence of serious hepatotoxity. (It is noteworthy, however, that the development of two other thiazolidinediones—ciglitazone and englitazone—was discontinued because of adverse hepatic effects.) In contrast to troglitazone, rosiglitazone does not appear to induce the CYP 3A4 system of cytochrome P450; this may reduce the potential for interactions during combination therapy with other antidiabetic agents. Increases in lactate dehydrogenase and creatine kinase have occasionally been observed during pioglitazone therapy. However, no drug interactions have been reported

Table 3.7 Pharmacokinetic features of the thiazolidinediones rosiglitazone and pioglitazone.

	Rosiglitazone	Pioglitazone
Time to peak plasma concentration	~1 h	< 2 h
Plasma t$_{1/2}$	~3.5 h*	3–7 h*
Plasma protein-bound	> 99%	> 99%
Hepatic metabolism	Mainly via CYP2C8 to weakly active metabolites	Mainly via CYP2C8 to active metabolites
Elimination	Mainly urine	Mainly bile

* Longer if metabolites included. Adapted from Krentz, A.J. & Bailey, C.J. 2001. Reproduced with permission from Krentz, A.J. & Bailey, C.J. 2001. *Type 2 Diabetes in Practice*. Royal Society of Medicine Press, London.

with this agent either. The pharmacokinetic features of rosiglitazone and pioglitazone are presented in Table 3.7

Weight gain

Increases of up to 2 kg were reported in clinical trials of troglitazone. Reduced glycosuria consequent upon improved glycaemic control may have been contributory but other factors have been suggested including the improvement in insulin sensitivity in lipid metabolism which favours lipogenesis.

Weight gain appears to have be maximal during the initial weeks of therapy, plateauing thereafter. In a 12 week study troglitazone monotherapy was associated with a reduction in intra-abdominal fat mass, no significant overall change in body weight being observed. In another study, weight gain during troglitazone therapy was in subcutaneous rather than intra-abdominal depots. These observations are of interest in view of the reported association between abdominal adiposity and insulin resistance. Site-specific activation of PPAR-γ has been reported in human pre-adipocytes. Thus, omental cells are refractory to stimulation of PPAR-γ by thiazolidinediones, contrasting with the actions of these agents in subcutaneous pre-adipocytes. Weight gain has also been reported in clinical studies of rosiglitazone and pioglitazone averaging approximately 3 kg at 26 weeks for the former agent. The risk

Weight gain is an adverse effect of thiazolidinediones

is somewhat higher when the drugs are combined with sulphonylureas.

Cardiovascular and haemodynamic effects

Preclinical studies suggested the potential hazards of haemodilution, fluid retention, cardiomegaly and anaemia. With the exception of oedema and mild anaemia (usually very minor) in patients treated with troglitazone or rosiglitazone, these have not been considered to be major clinical importance. However, in Europe rosglitazone and pioglitazone are contraindicated in patients with any degree of heart failure. Patients with impaired cardiac reserve should be monitored closely. A higher incidence of cardiac failure was noted in trials which combined rosiglitazone with insulin. Reports of a potentially advantageous blood pressure-lowering effect have not been evident in all studies. In view of the putative relationship between insulin resistance and hypertension, both of which are prominent features of type 2 diabetes, this observation merits further study. It is hypothesized that thiazolidinediones reduce blood pressure via effects on vascular calcium channels.

Rosiglitazone and pioglitazone are contra-indicated in patients with cardiac failure

Hypoglycaemia

This is a risk when thiazolidinediones are combined with other agents such as sulphonylureas or insulin; careful monitoring of blood glucose is required and insulin doses may have to be reduced, sometimes substantially. There should be no risk of hypoglaecemia in combination with metformin since neither agent causes hypoglaecemia as non-therapy.

Fertility

In pre-menopausal women with hyperinsulinaemia-associated anovulation, treatment with insulin-sensitizing agents may restore fertility (Section 2.5.12). Thus, such patients may be warned of the risk of pregnancy.

Anti-atherogenic effects

Animal models suggest anti-atherogenic effects of thiazolidinediones. In view of their beneficial effects on components of the metabolic syndrome, pioglitazone and rosiglitazone are being studied in trials with cardiovascular end-points.

3.2.3 Sulphonylureas

Extensive experience has been built with sulphonylureas in type 2 diabetes since their introduction in the 1950s. However, uncertainties about cardiovascular safety of these drugs, raised by the UGDP in the 1970s, persist.

Clinical indications

As sulphonylureas lower blood glucose in patients with type 2 diabetes by stimulating insulin secretion, they are indicated in patients for whom relative insulin deficiency —rather than insulin resistance—is thought to be the predominant biochemical abnormality. Because measurement of insulin sensitivity is not possible in routine practice this requires clinical judgement. Patients with obesity are more appropriate candidates for metformin or thiazolidinediones; the neutral effects of metformin on body weight make this drug the treatment of choice. Weight gain with sulphonylureas is well recognized. In the UKPDS, glibenclamide-treated patients gained an additional 1.7 kg and chlorpropamide-treated patients 2.6 kg above the weight gained by the diet-only group.

Mode of action

Insulin secretion
Sulphonylureas lower blood glucose (even in non-diabetics) primarily by stimulating insulin secretion from the islet β-cells. This is accomplished by binding to specific cellular receptors resulting in closure of membrane ATP-dependent potassium channels. This, in turn, causes depolarization, entry of calcium ions and, ultimately, exocytosis of insulin granules.

Extra-pancreatic effects
The contribution of direct extra-pancreatic effects to glucose lowering has long been debated, the generally accepted view being that these are of marginal importance. *In vivo* studies have not been able to distinguish between direct tissue effects and indirect effects produced by reversal of glucotoxicity or lipotoxicity (see Section 1.6.2).

However, the recently introduced long-acting sulphonylurea, glimepiride, facilitates translocation of GLUT-1 and GLUT-4 glucose transporters in insulin-resistant adipocytes *in vitro*. Moreover, *in vivo* studies indicate that glimepiride, which binds predominantly to a different part of the sulphonylurea receptor, may attain equivalent blood glucose control with less hyperinsulinaemia than agents such as glibenclamide. Enhanced insulin sensitivity might account for this observation. There are reports that weight gain may also be less pronounced with this agent than is usual with other sulphonylureas; this requires confirmation.

Cardiovascular safety

The high incidence of coronary events in patients with type 2 diabetes (allied to a worse outcome than for non-diabetics) demands that the cardiovascular safety of antidiabetic drugs is beyond question. Unfortunately, despite years of controversy this issue remains shrouded in uncertainty. In the UGDP patients allocated to the sulphonylurea, tolbutamide (or phenformin), fared less well than patients treated with diet or insulin. Criticisms of the design and analysis of this trial, allied to results from studies suggesting a cardioprotective effect of sulphonylureas, led to widespread rejection of the findings in Europe. The weight gain and hyperinsulinaemia associated with sulphonylureas have been regarded as undesirable but these effects may be countered by cardioprotective improvements in glycaemia, lipids, and fibrinolysis induced by sulphonylureas.

More recently, the debate has centred on the potentially adverse effects of closure of ATP-dependent potassium channels, which are not only present in the β-cells but also in the mitochondria of cardiomyocytes and vascular smooth muscle cells. Glibenclamide has been shown to inhibit cardioprotective ischaemic preconditioning in animal and human studies. However, many of these acute studies have used drug concentrations far in excess of those used therapeutically. The clinical implications of this effect, thought to be mediated via effects on vascular ATP-dependent potassium channels, remain uncertain. Differences between sulphonylureas on their vascular effects have been reported. Molecular studies indicate that

Some sulphonylureas close vascular ATP-dependent potassium channels gliclazide interacts specifically with the β-cell ATP-dependent potassium channel whereas glibenclamide (which also contains a bezamido moiety) blocks cardiac potassium channels as well. Glimepiride appears to be more selective for the islet ATP-dependent potassium channel than glibenclamide. Thus when administered acutely to non-diabetic humans glimepiride, in contrast to glibenclamide, appears not to inhibit ischaemic preconditioning.

Long-term clinical trials will be necessary to resolve the issue of the relative cardiovascular safety of different sulphonylureas. However, treatment with sulphonylureas emerged as a factor associated with a worse outcome following percutaneous transluminal coronary angioplasty in a *post hoc* analysis of the Bypass Angioplasty Revascularization Investigation (BARI) study. Moreover, in the Diabetes Mellitus Insulin Glucose Infusion in Acute Myocardial Infarction (DIGAMI) study, patients not receiving insulin on admission with an acute myocardial infarction showed the greatest benefit from intensive insulin therapy (see Section 2.6.1). This has led to speculation about whether withdrawal of sulphonylureas contributed to the improved outcome.

Many theoretical benefits of insulin therapy in acute coronary ischaemia may be invoked, including reduced myocardial utilization of fatty acids which may increase infarct size and favourable longer term metabolic effects. Finally, in the UKPDS, chlorpropamide therapy was associated with higher blood pressure and less effect on microvascular complications than glibenclamide; chloropropamide is now regarded as an obsolete drug.

In the DIGAMI study, intensive insulin therapy reduced mortality in diabetics following myocardial infarction

3.2.4 Meglitinide analogues

Repaglinide is a member of a new group of secretagogues, the meglitinide analogues (Fig. 3.9). Meglitinide is a benzoic acid derivative, being the non-sulphonylurea part of the glibenclamide molecule. Another agent in this class, mitiglinide, is in phase III clinical trials. Repaglininde binds to the ATP-dependent potassium channel at a site distinct from the sulphonylureas. Furthermore, in contrast to glibenclamide, repaglinide does not enter the β-cell to stimulate exocytosis of insulin-containing secretory

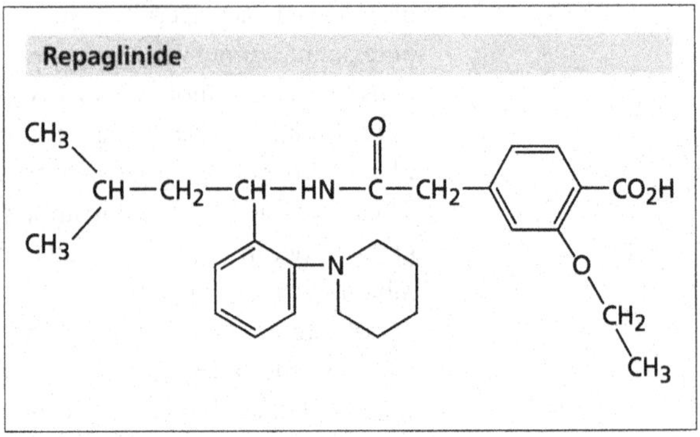

Fig. 3.9 Structure of repaglinide.

granules. Repaglinide requires the presence of glucose, in contrast to sulphonylureas which will stimulate insulin release in the absence of glucose. Repaglinide is effective when used as both monotherapy and in combination with metformin. The use of repaglinide in combination with troglitazone has also been investigated; preliminary reports suggest that combination therapy may be more effective than either drug when used as monotherapy. To date there have been no reports of studies specifically examining the effect of repaglinide on insulin sensitivity in humans.

Repaglinide is taken with meals with the aim of controlling post-prandial hyperglycaemia; if no meal is consumed the corresponding dose is omitted. In placebo-controlled clinical trials, reductions in post-prandial glucose approaching 6 mmol/L have been reported. Significant decreases in fasting plasma glucose and glycated haemoglobin (HbA_{1c}) concentrations have also been observed. Repaglinide is rapidly absorbed, reaching peak plasma levels in less than 1 h and is rapidly excreted (90%) via the liver. Starting dosage is 0.5 mg (or 1 mg if transferring from another sulphonylurea) titrated upwards at 1- to 2-week intervals to a maximum single dose of 4 mg with main meals; total maximum dose 16 mg/day. Repaglinide is generally well-tolerated with only minor adverse events; no significant drug interactions have been reported. Data showing a lower risk of hypoglycaemia when compared with sulphonylureas would make it an attractive option for older patients at highest risk. The drug is also a safe choice in

Repaglinide is used principally as a short-acting prandial glucose regulator patients with impaired renal function. However, to date there is limited experience with the drug.

Although often considered alongside repaglinide, nateglinide is a D-phenylalanine derivative. Nateglinide has an even shorter duration of binding to the islet β-cell. Nateglinide was launched in the UK in 2001 and is presently licensed for use only in combination with metformin. As with repaglinide, the reported risks of hypoglycaemia and weight gain appear to be reduced compared with some sulphonylureas. Other novel insulin secretoagogues the have been considered for possible use in type 2 diabetes include succinate esters, morpholinoguanidines, imidazolines, glucagon-like peptide-1 and exendin-4.

3.2.5 α-Glucosidase inhibitors

Acarbose

With repaglinide and nateglinide, acarbose is considered to be a member of the 'prandial glucose regulators'. Acarbose, a pseudotetrasaccharide and the most established agent in this class, reduces the rate of carbohydrate absorption from the gastrointestinal tract by inhibiting the action of the enzyme complex α-glucosidase in the brush border of the small intestine; post-prandial increases in blood glucose are thereby reduced (Fig. 3.10). Enhanced secretion of the incretin hormone glucagon-like peptide-1 from the small intestine may represent an additional mode of action.

In a study of patients with impaired glucose tolerance, acarbose 100 mg t.d.s. decreased post-prandial plasma glucose and insulin concentrations and improved insulin sensitivity as assessed using the insulin suppression test. However, no significant improvement in insulin sensitivity has been demonstrated in studies of patients with established type 2 diabetes using the glucose clamp technique.

Serious adverse effects of acarbose are rare; systemic absorption of the parent drug and its metabolites is low. Hypoglycaemia is not a risk if the drug is used as monotherapy. However, tolerability is limited by gastrointestinal side-effects (flatulence, diarrhoea and abdominal pain); the latter requires introduction at low doses and careful dose titration. Most patients withdraw from therapy during the

Acabose reduces post-prandial glucose and insulin concentrations and can improve sensitivity

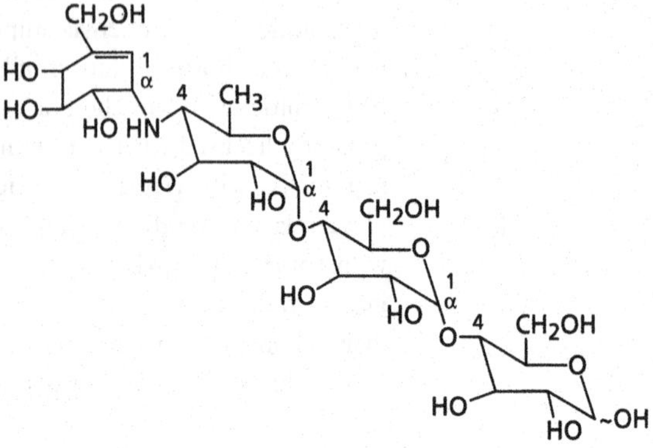

Fig. 3.10 Structure of acarbose.

early stages. If tolerance can be established, continued therapy may be more easily sustained. Increases in plasma concentrations of hepatic transaminases have been reported at higher doses; isolated cases of more severe hepatotoxicity have also been described. However, the drug is neutral with respect to effects on body weight.

Clinical studies have generally demonstrated lower efficacy of acarbose compared with sulphonylureas or biguanides. Acarbose may be combined with either sulphonylureas, metformin or insulin. In the UKPDS acarbose was added in later as a supplementary therapy, regardless of the original treatment allocation. On an intention-to-treat analysis, the reduction in HbA_{1c} was only 0.2%; however, in the minority of patients (39%) who were able to tolerate the drug a mean reduction in HbA_{1c} of 0.5% was observed (compared with placebo) at 3 years. Not all studies have demonstrated improvements in HbA_{1c} concentrations with acarbose.

Acarbose has a neutral effect on body weight

Miglitol

Another α-glucosidase inhibitor, miglitol, was launched in the USA in 1999. This is a competitive and reversible inhibitor with a shorter duration of action than acarbose. In contrast to acarbose, the drug is absorbed and excreted unchanged by the kidneys. Reductions in post-prandial hyperglycaemia have been reported in patients with type 2 diabetes. Miglitol may be usefully combined with sulphonylureas. As is the case for acarbose, miglitol is not associated with hypoglycaemia or weight-gain when used as monotherapy. The profile of gastrointestinal side-effects is similar to those encountered with acarbose (placebo-subtracted reductions in HbA_{1c} of 0.42 and 0.43%, respectively). However, several small trials have failed to show any significant improvements in insulin sensitivity with miglitol.

Voglibose

Voglibose, a potent inhibitor of sucrase, has been studied in patients with type 2 diabetes. In the same way as acarbose (see Section 3.2.5), voglibose reportedly stimulates release of the incretin glucagon-like peptide-1 from the intestine. There is no evidence to date for an effect of voglibose on insulin sensitivity in humans.

3.2.6 Insulin

Insulin treatment is usually regarded as a therapy of last resort for many patients with type 2 diabetes. However, there are a number of clinical situations in which insulin is the treatment of choice, e.g. pregnancy.

Insulin therapy is often regarded as a treatment of last resort for patients with type 2 diabetes

Contraindications or failure to respond to oral antidiabetic agents may necessitate early use of insulin. However, most patients with type 2 diabetes receiving long-term insulin treatment do so because oral agents, even in combination, have ultimately failed to produce adequate glycaemic control (often termed 'secondary failure'). Reluctance to use insulin earlier in such patients derives from the mode of delivery and unwanted effects of insulin. In addition to the inconvenience of insulin treatment (and the blood glucose monitoring which accompanies it), insulin treatment is associated with weight gain and risk of hypoglycaemia. There have also been concerns that exogenous insulin treatment might accelerate atherogenesis (see Section 2.5). However, weight gain is not inevitable (and may be limited by concomitant use of metformin) and the risk of severe hypoglycaemia is very much lower than for

Insulin treatment is often associated with weight gain in patients with type 2 diabetes

patients with type 1 diabetes. Moreover, patients often derive symptomatic benefit when transferred to insulin and quality of life may not be impaired. Recent studies have demonstrated that intensive insulin therapy can be a safe and efficacious therapeutic option for selected patients with type 2 diabetes. Insulin therapy may also improve insulin-sensitivity via control of hyperglycaemia.

United Kingdom Prospective Diabetes Study

The UKPDS included groups of normal weight and over-weight patients who were randomized to insulin mono-therapy if initial dietary measures proved insufficient. Although insulin treatment failed to prevent a progressive rise in glucose levels over 15 years (Fig. 3.3) and led to a mean weight gain 4 kg in excess of the diet-treatment control group it successfully reduced diabetes-related end-points via improved glycaemic control. The annual incidence of major hypoglycaemia was 1.8% (compared with 1.4% for glibenclamide). Importantly, there was no evidence that insulin increased the incidence of macro-vascular complications. Thus, insulin is increasingly being viewed as an appropriate and safe therapy for patients with type 2 diabetes. The introduction of insulin analogues (see below) and improved insulin delivery systems (including the pulmonary route) may further increase the acceptability of insulin treatment.

Insulin as monotherapy

Twice-daily insulin, conventionally administered as isophane (neutral protamine hagedorn, NPH) or premixed prepara-tions (e.g. 30% short-acting, 70% isophane or in 50 : 50 com-bination), is often effective in patients with type 2 diabetes. Pen injectors may improve acceptability and compliance, although elderly patients may experience practical difficult-ies resulting from limited dexterity or visual impairment. The pharmacokinetics of isophane insulin are such that once-daily injections will rarely produce glycaemic control that is satisfactory throughout the day. In particular, adequate suppression of overnight endogenous glucose production is necessary to control fasting hyperglycaemia. Insulin-mediated suppression of plasma fatty-acid concentrations may contribute to reductions in hepatic glucose production. Longer-acting insulins, e.g. ultralente, have been used as the basis of regimens wherein the long-acting preparation provides background (basal) low-level insulin upon which premeal boluses of short-acting insulin are superimposed. Such regimens are not used extensively in patients with type 2 diabetes. This applies to other strategies, such as pump-delivered continuous subcutaneous insulin infusions. Currently available long-acting insulins, such as ultralente, do not provide stable plasma levels of insulin; analogues (e.g. insulin glargine) with improved pharmacokinetics offer advantages including reduced rates of hypoglycaemia.

Combination therapy using insulin and oral agents

Combining
insulin with oral
antidiabetic
agents may be
advantageous

Several studies have suggested that combination therapy using insulin with either sulphonylureas, metformin or thiazolidinediones may be advantageous. Although detractors voice concerns about polypharmacy, the clinical and biochemical heterogeneity of type 2 diabetes suggests that there may be merit in tailoring treatment to the individual. With an expanding range of oral agents this approach may become more popular.

Insulin and sulphonylureas

Clinical trials have demonstrated reduced insulin requirements and less marked weight gain when sulphonylureas are combined with insulin. Daytime sulphonylurea therapy with a morning or evening injection of isophane (NPH) insulin provides comparable short-term glycaemic control to two daily injections of premixed insulin. However, it is uncertain whether advantages in terms of weight gain described for sulphonylurea plus evening insulin are independent of improvements in glycaemic control. Residual endogenous insulin secretion is a prerequisite for successful combination therapy.

Insulin and metformin

There is some evidence for less marked weight gain when insulin is combined with metformin. In a recent randomized controlled trial in patients with secondary failure of

159

sulphonylureas, metformin plus bedtime insulin has provided the best glycaemic control and the lowest rate of hypoglycaemia in concert with negligible weight gain during 12 months follow-up. Less dramatic benefits are generally the case in clinical practice.

Insulin and thiazolidinediones

The introduction of troglitazone, rosiglitazone and pioglitazone has added another class of agents which may be usefully combined with insulin. Glycaemic control may be improved, thereby allowing a reduction in insulin dose. However, the long-term gains from this approach are uncertain.

3.3 Antiobesity drugs

Drug therapy for obesity is regarded as an adjunct to diet and lifestyle measures; as the latter are generally safe manoeuvres, drug-associated toxicity is a crucial issue in the management of obesity. In 1997 reports of cardiac valve lesions led to the withdrawal of the amphetamine-related anorectic agents fenfluramine (often used in combination with phenteramine in the USA) and dexfenfluramine.

Dexfenfluramine was withdrawn following reports of heart valve lesions.

There is some evidence that dexfenfluramine possesses insulin-sensitizing properties. Chronic therapy ameliorated hepatic and peripheral tissue insulin resistance in animal studies; limited human studies suggest effects on insulin action independent of changes in body weight. Notwithstanding these problems of toxicity, the potentially lucrative and expanding market for antiobesity drugs continues to stimulate new developments. Several other drugs are under consideration as satiety factors. However, the redundancy of molecular mechanisms regulating body weight cautions against a single effective pharmacological solution.

3.3.1 Sibutramine

Sibutramine is a serotonin and noradrenaline neuronal reuptake inhibitor, licensed currently in the USA and some other countries. Sibutramine is a more selective inhibitor of serotonin reuptake than fenfluramine and dexfenfluramine. It reduces appetite while also producing small increases in energy expenditure via increased thermogenesis. Small increases in blood pressure (an effect also observed with phentermine) and heart rate have been reported, indicating the need for careful monitoring. Sibutramine is contra-indicated in patients with ischaemic heart disease. However, there have no reports of cardiac valve lesions to date. Improved metabolic control has been reported in type 2 diabetes. Favourable effects on HDL-cholesterol and triglycerides were reported in a recent placebo-controlled trial over 24 months in non-diabetic subjects.

3.3.2 Orlistat

Orlistat is a pancreatic lipase inhibitor which inhibits triglyceride digestion. Undigested fat is excreted un-changed leading to a moderately high incidence of pre-dictable side-effects including abdominal pains, flatulence, oily spotting, diarrhoea and urgency. It has been suggested that these side-effects may encourage compliance with a reduced-fat diet. The use of orlistat doubles the mean weight loss (approximately 10% body weight) obtained with diet alone after 12 months of treatment.

Orlistat doubles the weight loss achieved with diet alone

Improvements in glycaemia, total- and LDL-cholesterol concentrations and apoproteins have been reported in patients with obesity-related type 2 diabetes; the beneficial effects on lipids may be mediated in part by the reduction in dietary fat absorption. Serum insulin concentrations also decline modestly with longer term treatment (Fig. 3.11). Orlistat is licensed for use in patients with obesity (defined as a body mass index > 30 kg/m²) or in overweight patients (> 28 kg/m²) with additional cardiovascular risk factors. UK guidance requires that patients should have achieved weight loss of 2.5 kg prior to introduction of the drug; if subsequent weight loss is less than 5% of body weight ther-apy should be withdrawn.

Orlistat improves glycaemia and lipids in obese patients with type 2 diabetes

3.3.3 Leptin

Administration of leptin to obese or diabetic rodents im-proves sensitivity to insulin and reduces hyperinsulinaemia before changes in body weight are observed. However, lep-tin does not directly stimulate glucose disposal in muscle or adipose tissues; leptin-induced increases in fatty-acid oxida-

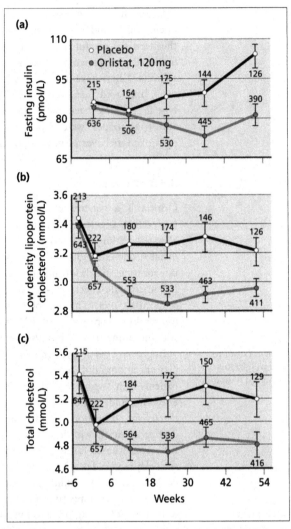

Fig. 3.11 Effects of orlistat in obese patients with type 2 diabetes. (a) Mean (±SE) fasting serum insulin concentrations; (b) fasting serum low-density lipoprotein cholesterol levels ($P < 0.05$ for placebo vs. orlistat); and (c) total cholesterol. Numbers above plot points are the numbers of patients. To convert to mU/L, + 6.0. (Redrawn from Davidson, M.H. *et al.* 1999. *Journal of the American Medical Association* **281**, 235–242.) To convert mmol/L to mg/dL, divide by 0.02586.

tion have been postulated. Other theoretical mechanisms include indirect effects mediated via the brain and sympathetic nervous system, increased levels of physical activity or enhanced thermogenesis. Administration of exogenous leptin produced dramatic reductions in hyperphagia and obesity in a child with congenital leptin deficiency. However, the role of leptin supplementation in the management of common forms of human obesity remains uncertain.

3.3.4 β_3-adrenocepter agonists

To date, these agents have had only limited success. Adrenergic side-effects have been a problem. Improvements in insulin action have been reported. However, there is potential for stimulation of lipolysis.

3.4 Lipid-modifying drugs

3.4.1 Fibric acid derivatives

This class of drugs is indicated mainly for mixed dyslipidaemias, i.e. where hypertriglyceridaemia or low HDL-cholesterol levels coexist with elevated total- or LDL-cholesterol concentrations. This pattern of dyslipidaemia is commonly encountered in patients with the insulin-resistance syndrome, including patients with type 2 diabetes (see Section 2.5.7). Evidence for efficacy of fibrates in preventing coronary events is presently less extensive than for statins. However, the Veterans Affairs High-density Lipoprotein Cholesterol Intervention Trial (VA-HIT) demonstrated a 22% relative reduction in risk ($P < 0.006$) in coronary deaths in men (25% of whom were diabetic) with coronary heart disease treated with gemfibrozil. In addition, the Diabetes Atherosclerosis Intervention Study (DAIS) showed a reduction in angiographic coronary lesions with fenofibrate in patients with type 2 diabetes. Studies are in progress to define which patients are most suitable for treatment with fibrates. Fibric acid derivatives have a multiplicity of effects on lipid metabolism including:

• Enhanced activity of lipoprotein lipase in adipose tissue and skeletal muscle leading to hydrolysis of triglyceride-rich lipoproteins.

- Decreases in the synthesis of apoprotein C-III—the major inhibitor of lipoprotein lipase.
- Reduction in the hepatic secretion of very low density lipoprotein (VLDL).
- Increased LDL catabolism.
- Increased cholesterol secretion into bile.
- Increased apoprotein A1 production (the major protein of HDL).

These effects appear to result from activation of peroxisome proliferator-activator receptor-α (cf. PPAR-γ, the principal target for thiazolidinediones). The tendency for plasma homocysteine levels to increase during fibrate therapy is potentially disadvantageous but of uncertain clinical significance. Fibric acid derivatives have been studied in patients with type 2 diabetes with the objective of improving glycaemic control. Fibrates lower plasma fatty-acid concentrations thereby reducing potential competition with glucose for uptake and oxidation (Randle cycle; see Section 1). However, the effects of fibrates on glycaemic control are generally minor. Much more impressive results have been reported in patients with lipodystrophic diabetes (see Section 2.4). Fibrates may sometimes have dramatic effects on glycaemic control and insulin sensitivity in such patients if major disturbances of lipid metabolism are also evident. Fibrates should be avoided in renal failure.

> Fibrates can produce major improvements in glucose and lipid metabolism in patients with lipodystrophy

3.4.2 Acipimox

Acipimox is a long-acting analogue of nicotinic acid which suppresses lipolysis thereby lowering plasma fatty-acid concentrations. The short duration of action of nicotinic acid results in rebound elevations of fatty acids and a deterioration in glucose tolerance. Although not all studies with acipimox have shown effects on insulin sensitivity, a twofold overall increase in insulin-stimulated glucose uptake was observed in lean and obese patients with or without impaired glucose tolerance or type 2 diabetes (Fig. 3.12). In the latter study, three doses of acipimox were administered overnight to maximize suppression of fatty acids. Improvements of ~ 30% were observed in the curves for glucose and insulin during 75 oral glucose tolerance tests.

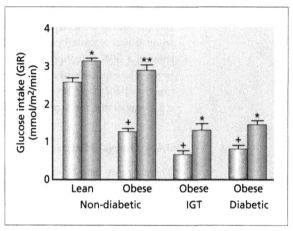

Fig. 3.12 Rates of glucose infusion required to maintain euglycaemia during hyperinsulinaemic clamps in lean and obese non-diabetic subjects and in patients with impaired glucose tolerance (IGT) or type 2 diabetes after overnight treatment with placebo (light bars) or acipimox (dark bars). $*P < 0.001$, $**P < 0.0001$ for placebo vs. Acipimuox $+P < 0.001$ vs. Lean non-diabetic controls. (Reproduced with permission from Santomauro, A.T.M.G. *et al.* 1999. *Diabetes* **48**, 1836–1841.) GIR, glucose infusion rate.

3.4.3 Statins

Inihibitors of the rate-limiting enzyme of cholesterol synthesis (hydroxy methyl glutaryl coenzyme A reductase) are used extensively to reduce cardiovascular risk. Their application is likely to expand with publication of the Heart Protection Study. This showed significant reductions in events in numerous high-risk groups, including patients with type 2 diabetes, using simvastatin. The principal action of this class of agents is to lower LDL-cholesterol levels. In addition, reductions in triglycerides and effects on endothelial function have been reported. Data concerning effects of statins on insulin sensitivity, however, are scant. In a double-blind cross-over study, simvastatin 30 mg improved insulin-mediated glucose disposal and enhanced suppression of hepatic glucose production in elderly patients with type 2 diabetes, reduced plasma non-esterified fatty-acid concentrations being implicated. However other investigators have not confirmed a beneficial effect of simvastatin on insulin sensitivity using the euglycaemic clamp technique. Recent data from the West of Scotland study using pravastatin as a primary prevention therapy showed a 30% reduction in incident cases of type 2 diabetes. The mechanisms are uncertain; effects on cytokines (Section 1.6.2) have been suggested. More potent statins, e.g. rosuvastatin, are currently in development.

3.4.4 Omega-3 fatty acids

These agents may be useful in the treatment of severe hypertriglyceridaemia. However, large doses may be required which can impair glycaemic control in patients with type 2 diabetes. Increases in plasma LDL-cholesterol concentrations have also been reported. Benefits of fish oils have been shown in (mainly non-diabetic) survivors of myocardial infarction.

3.5 Antihypertensive drugs

Hypertension is more prevalent in patients with type 2 diabetes (see Section 2.5.6). The UKPDS included a blood pressure substudy (Hypertension in Diabetes Study; HDS) which showed clear benefits of tight control (mean 144/82 vs. 154/87 mmHg) of hypertension. The following statistically significant benefits were observed from tight control:

- 32% reduction in diabetes-related deaths.
- 34% reduction in progression of diabetic retinopathy.
- 37% reduction in microvascular complications.
- 44% reduction in non-fatal stroke.
- 66% reduction in cardiac failure.

This study also compared atenolol and captopril as main therapies (see below). No significant difference was observed in the effects of these agents. However, most patients required two or more drugs to attain blood-pressure control. Other major hypertension studies in recent years have included diabetic subgroups (Table 3.8). Each of these has shown considerable benefits for diabetic patients in reducing cardiovascular events. The magnitude of the benefit has tended to be greater for diabetic patients than for the non-diabetics, reflecting the higher absolute risk associated with diabetes.

The Hypertension in Diabetes Study showed major benefits from tight blood pressure control in type 2 diabetes

Table 3.8 Randomized hypertension trials that have included patients with type 2 diabetes.

> **1** *Systolic Hypertension in the Elderly Program (SHEP)**
> Total *n* = 4736; diabetic *n* = 583
> Chlorthalidone ± atenolol or reserpine
> *Findings.* Reduction in major cardiovascular events (cerebral and cardiac) with active treatment vs. placebo. Greater benefit in diabetic subgroup reflecting higher absolute risk
>
> **2** *Hypertension Optimal Treatment trial (HOT)†*
> Total *n* = 18 790; diabetic *n* = 1501
> Felodipine + other agents as required to attain blood pressure targets
> *Findings.* Reduction (by 50%) in major cardiovascular events with target diastolic of 80 mmHg vs. 90 mmHg in diabetic patients
>
> **3** *SYST-EUR‡*
> Total *n* = 4695; diabetic *n* = 492
> Nitrendipine + enalapril or thiazide
> *Findings.* Excess risk of diabetes almost completely eliminated by antihypertensive therapy with major reductions (approx 70%) in cardiovascular mortality and all cardiovascular end-points

* *Journal of the American Medical Association* 1996; **276**, 1886–1892.
† *Lancet* 1998; **351**, 1755–1762.
‡ *Lancet* 1997; **350**, 757–764 and *New England Journal of Medicine* 1999; **340**, 677–684.

3.5.1 β-Adrenergic blockers and thiazide diuretics

For many years, controversy has surrounded the effects of these antihypertensive agents on risk factors for cardiovascular disease. While the clinical significance of these effects remains uncertain, treatment of hypertension has not produced the expected reduction in mortality from coronary heart disease in trials using β-blockers and thiazides. It has been suggested that adverse metabolic effects might have offset the beneficial effects of these drugs. However, recent trial data suggest that the reduction in cardiovascular events using regimens based on these agents is similar to newer agents. Adverse metabolic effects include the following.

Non-selective β-blockers and high-dose thiazides impair insulin sensitivity

• *Insulin action.* β-Blockers (particularly non-selective agents) and high-dose thiazide diuretics may aggravate insulin resistance. In a double-blind cross-over trial, 5.0 mg/day bendrofluazide increased hepatic glucose production and fasting serum insulin concentration. By contrast, 1.25 mg/day was equally effective in lowering blood pressure and was devoid of any adverse metabolic effects.

• In the HDS, mean HbA_{1c} in atenolol-treated patients was significantly higher than that for captopril-treated patients during the first few years of the study; more anti-hyperglycaemic therapy was required in the atenolol-treated patients. Moreover, both β-blockers and thiazides, particularly in combination, have been implicated in the pathogenesis of type 2 diabetes in patients with essential hypertension during longitudinal studies. However, it has not been determined whether this effect reflects adverse effects on insulin sensitivity. Cardevilol has both non-selective (β- and $α_1$-blocking activity). In a randomized comparative trial in non-diabetic hypertensive patients, insulin sensitivity during glucose clamps increased, whereas it declined with the $β_1$-selective agent, metoprolol.

• *Lipids.* The adverse effect of these agents on plasma lipids (increased very-low-density lipoproteins and hypercholesterolaemia, respectively) has also received attention. Associated haemostatic abnormalities (increased fibrinogen and factor VII, reduced activity of plasminogen activator inhibitor-1) may contribute to atherogenesis.

• *Hypokalaemia.* There have been reports of increased risk of sudden death in diabetic and non-diabetic patients with electrocardiographic abnormalities treated with thiazides.

The metabolic effects of thiazides can be minimized by the use of low doses. Doses higher than 2.5 mg/day bendrofluazide have limited additional antihypertensive effect and increase the risk of adverse effects. There is now clear evidence from clinical trials that thiazide-based treatment is particularly beneficial in patients with diabetes. Thus any adverse metabolic effects appear to be outweighed by the benefits of reducing blood pressure.

3.5.2 Calcium-channel blockers

Dihydropyridine calcium antagonists with a short duration of action, e.g. nifedipine, may also impair insulin action. However, longer-acting drugs (e.g. amlodipine) and modified release nifedepine, together with non-dihydropyridine drugs (e.g. diltiazem, verapamil) appear to have neutral effects. Calcium-channel blockers (felodipine and nitrendepine) significantly reduced cardiovascular events in trials involving hypertensive patients with type 2 diabetes (see Table 3.8). However, concerns have been expressed that some recent trials have shown inferiority of calcium-channel blockers compared with other agents. Two recent comparative studies, in which calcium-channel blockers have been compared with diuretics and β-blockers have shown similar efficacy.

Long-acting calcium-channel blockers have neutral effects on insulin sensitivity

3.5.3 Angiotensin converting enzyme inhibitors

The effects of ACE inhibitors on insulin sensitivity remains controversial

These agents are either neutral or possibly may improve insulin sensitivity in non-diabetic and diabetic patients; however, the design of some human studies purporting to demonstrate improved insulin action has attracted criticism.

Angiotensin converting enzyme gene polymorphisms may have implications for effects on insulin action in addition to therapeutic responses to angiotensin converting enzyme inhibitors. Captopril improves insulin-mediated glucose transport in the obese Zucker rat. Imidapril increases phosphatidylinositol-3-kinase activity and tissue blood flow in Zucker fatty rats. In hypertensive humans with abdominal obesity, enalapril improves the sensitivity of lipolysis to insulin. Both captopril and ramipril have been shown to reduce vascular complications in clinical trials of patients with diabetes. The Heart Outcomes Prevention Evaluation (HOPE, see Section 3.1.1) provided strong support for use of ramipril in high-risk patients with type 2 diabetes. Hypertension was not a prerequisite for entry into the latter study. Compared with placebo, ramipril produced significant reductions in diabetes-related complications. The diabetic subgroup shared the reduction in cardiovascular events observed in the total cohort. Moreover, in accordance with some other studies, the incidence of self-reported new cases of diabetes was significantly reduced in ramipril-treated patients (relative risk 0.68, $P = 0.002$). This finding is being examined further in a new study. Of theoretical interest is the fact that the renin–angiotensin system is present in the endocrine pancreas.

3.5.4 Angiotensin II receptor antagonists

There are reports of improved insulin action with these agents in animal models and human studies. Losartan improves glucose tolerance and insulin sensitivity in the fructose-fed rat. Angiotensin II (subtype-1) receptor antagonists block cross-talk between insulin and the angiotensin II receptor. Losartan and inbesartan have protective effects in patients with type 2 diabetes and nephropathy.

3.5.5 α_1-Receptor blockers

Some α_1-blockers have favourable effects on insulin sensitivity and lipids

Doxazosin has been shown to improve insulin sensitivity, glucose tolerance and plasma lipid profiles in hypertensive patients with type 2 diabetes. Decreases in plasma plasminogen activator inhibitor-1 have also been reported. Thus, doxazosin ameliorates several components of the insulin-resistance syndrome.

3.5.6 Selective imidazoline receptor agonists

These centrally-acting sympatholytic agents lower blood pressure and may have beneficial effects on other aspects of the insulin-resistance syndrome. Moxonidine improves insulin action and lowers fatty acid concentrations in animal models of insulin resistance. In a placebo-controlled trial in obese hypertensive patients moxonidine 0.2 mg b.d. improved insulin-mediated glucose disposal in euglycaemic clamp studies; this effect was most evident in patients having the lowest insulin sensitivity index at baseline (Fig. 3.13) in whom insulin sensitivity improved by 21%. Fasting plasma glucose and insulin concentrations declined by approximately 5 and 10%, respectively, in the latter group.

Rilmenidine, another agent in this class, has also been shown to improve metabolic defects in insulin-resistant animals; effects on glucose and lipid metabolism in humans with diabetes appear to be neutral.

3.5.7 Aspirin

Aspirin is widely used in patients at high risk of cardiovascular events. Recent evidence shows that in addition to its

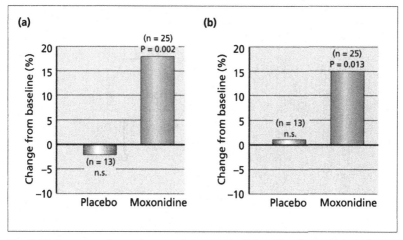

Fig. 3.13 Percentage changes in mean glucose uptake (M) and insulin sensitivity index (M/I) after 8 weeks' treatment with moxonidine 0.2 mg b.d. or placebo in patients with baseline M/I-values of 0–3.6. (Redrawn with permission from Haenni, A. & Lithell, H. 1999. *Journal of Hypertension* 17 (suppl. 3), S29–S35.)

antiplatelet effects, aspirin at high doses can also improve insulin signalling in experimental insulin resistance.

3.6 Experimental therapies

In addition to these agents, several classes of drugs with insulin-sensitizing actions are currently in various stages of development. Others have been evaluated but discarded as potential therapies. Some of these agents are considered briefly here.

3.6.1 D-*chiro*-inositol

The compound, D-*chiro*-inositol, has recently been proposed as a potential therapy for type 2 diabetes on the basis of studies in women with polycystic ovary syndrome (Fig. 3.14).

Based on the association between low tissue levels of *chiro*-inositol and insulin resistance, 44 obese women with polycystic ovary syndrome were treated with oral D-*chiro*-inositol (1200 mg/day) or placebo for 6–8 weeks. A significant reduction in insulin levels following oral glucose challenge was observed in the group of 22 women

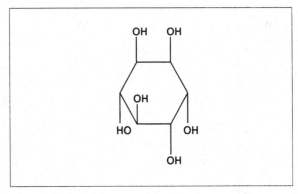

Fig. 3.14 Structure of D-*chiro* inositol.

who received D-*chiro*-inositol. This was accompanied by a significant decrease in plasma testosterone concentration, triglycerides and blood pressure, compared with placebo; no adverse effects were observed. In addition, 19 of the 22 women who received D-*chiro*-inositol ovulated as compared with two of the women in the placebo group. In support of this suggestion, in six women with impaired glucose tolerance at baseline, D-*chiro*-inositol significantly reduced the area under the plasma glucose curve, resulting in normal glucose tolerance; no significant improvement was noted in four similar women in the placebo group.

3.6.2 Non-thiazolidinedione PPAR-γ agonists

Members of this class of non-thiazolidinedione PPAR-γ agonists with insulin-sensitizing, lipid lowering and blood pressure-lowering properties are currently in phase III studies. No comparative studies with thiazolidinediones are available.

3.6.3 α-Lipoic acid

α-Lipoic (thioctic) acid is a potent lipophilic free radical scavenger which has been shown to improve glucose uptake in the muscle of insulin-resistant rodents and also to stimulate pyruvate dehydrogenase, thereby reducing plasma concentrations of the gluconeogenic precursors, lactate and pyruvate. In a study of patients with type 2 diabetes, using the modified frequently sampled intravenous glucose tolerance test, α-lipoic acid (600 mg b.d. for 4 weeks) reduced fasting blood plasma lactate and pyruvate concentrations which were elevated at baseline compared with levels in non-diabetic controls. An improvement in insulin sensitivity was observed in the lean subgroup of the diabetic patients, an improvement in glucose-effectiveness (regarded as reflecting the ability of glucose to promote its own disappearance from the circulation, see Section 1.5.4) being observed in both lean and overweight patients. However, as no treatment control group was included in this study these observations require confirmation.

3.6.4 Insulin-like growth factor-1

Recombinant insulin-like growth factor-1 has been used successfully in the treatment of ketoacidosis associated with rare conditions such as Rabson–Mendenhall syndrome (see Section 2.4) that are characterized by severe impairment of insulin action. Insulin-like growth factor-1 has also been evaluated as a potential treatment for type 2 diabetes but adverse clinical effects and mitogenic potential have hindered development.

3.6.5 Vanadium salts

A number of trace elements have been reported to exert insulin-like effects in muscle, liver and adipose tissue and enhance glucose metabolism independently of insulin. Of these, vanadium salts (e.g. bismalto-oxovanadium) have received the most attention. Vanadium activates serine/threonine kinases involved in intracellular insulin signalling at sites distal to the insulin receptor, thereby preventing protein dephosphorylation through inhibition of tyrosine phosphatases. Vanadium compounds also have an anorectic effect which may have contributed to glucose-lowering effects observed in certain animal models. Initial clinical trials have reported a beneficial effect in type 2 diabetes. However, the toxicity of vanadium is well recognized.

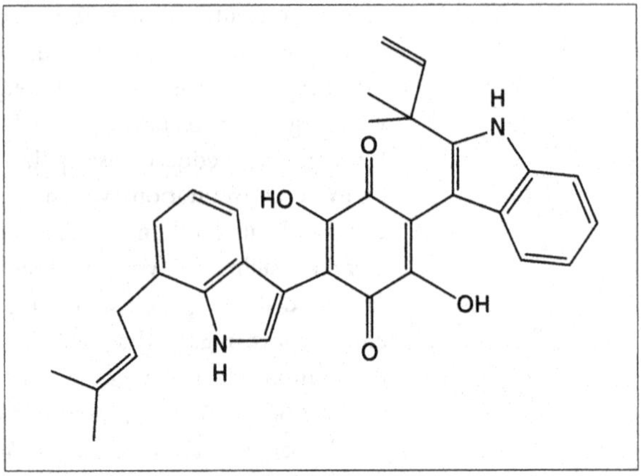

Fig. 3.15 Structure of a novel non-peptidyl fungal metabolite, L 738281, that is a selective agonist at insulin receptors. (Reproduced with permission from Zhang, B. *et al*. 1999. *Science* **284**, 9794–9797.)

3.6.6 The search for new drugs

In 1999, a novel non-peptidyl fungal metabolite (Fig. 3.15) was discovered which has insulin-mimetic activity in several biochemical and cellular assays. In contrast to vanadate, L 738281 is selective for the insulin receptor. Although it would be premature to speculate whether this discovery might lead to a novel class of antidiabetic agents, the compound was identified during a systematic search for molecules with insulin receptor-activating activity. Such approaches offer the possibility of advances in therapy for insulin resistance. However, recent experience with troglitazone madates careful testing for toxicity in the preclinical and clinical stages of development. Other therapeutic approaches have included inhibitors of fatty acid oxidation, glucose-6-phosphatase inhibitors and antagonists of glucagon. None have resulted in viable treatments to date.

3.7 Further reading

American Diabetes Association (1999) Nutrition recommendations and principles for people with diabetes mellitus. *Diabetes Care* **22** (Suppl. 1), S42–S45.

Ashcroft, F.M., Gribble, F.M. (1999) ATP-sensitive K+ channels and insulin secretion: their role in health and disease. *Diabetologia* **42**, 903–919.

Auwerx, J. (1999) PPAR-γ, the ultimate thrifty gene. *Diabetologica* **42**, 1033–1049.

Bailey, C.J. & Turner, R.C. (1996) Metformin. *New England Journal of Medicine* **334**, 574–579.

Barnett, A.H. (2001) Maximising outcomes in type 2 diabetes through weight management. *British Journal of Cardiology* **8**, 101–105.

Campbell, I. (1999) Repaglinide: a new short-acting hypoglycaemic agent. *Prescriber* **10**, 39–43.

Cusi, K. & DeFronzo, R.A. (1995) Treatment of NIDDM, IDDM, and other insulin-resistant states with IGF-1. *Diabetes Review* **3**, 206–236.

Day, C. (1999) Thiazolidinediones: a new class of oral antidiabetic drugs. *Diabetic Medicine* **16**, 179–192.

Diabetes Prevention Program Research Group (2002) Reduction in the incidence of type 2 diabetes with lifestyle intervention or metformin. *New England Journal of Medicine* **346**, 393–403.

Eriksson, J., Timela, S. & Koivisto, V.A. (1997) Exercise and the metabolic syndrome. *Diabetologia* **40**, 125–135.

Evans, A.J. & Krentz, A.J. (2000) Benefits and risks of transfer from oral antidiabetic agents to insulin in type 2 diabetes. In: *Drug treatment of type 2 diabetes* (ed. A.J. Krentz), pp. 85–101. ADIS International, Auckland.

Evans, A.J. & Krentz, A.J. (1999) Glimepiride: a new sulphonylurea. *Prescriber* **10**, 51–58.

Evans, A.J. & Krentz, A.J. (1999) Recent developments and emerging therapies for type 2 diabetes. *Drugs in Research and Development* 275–294.

Fisher, B.M. (1999) Interventional cardiology in people with diabetes. *Diabetic Medicine* **16**, 531–532.

Gaede, P., Vedel, P., Parving, H.-H. & Pedersen, O. (1999) Intensified multifactorial intervention in patients with type 2 diabetes mellitus and microalbuminuria: the Steno type 2 randomized study. *Lancet* **353**, 617–622.

Heart Outcomes Prevention Evaluation (HOPE) Study Investigators (2000) Effects of ramipril on cardiovascular and microvascular outcomes in people with diabetes mellitus: results of the HOPE and micro-HOPE substudy. *Lancet* **355**, 253–259.

Heart Outcomes Prevention Evaluation Study Investigators. (2000) Effects of an angiotensin-converting enzyme inhibitor, ramipril, on death from cardiovascular causes, myocardial infarction, and stroke in high-risk patients. *New England Journal of Medicine*.

Hu, F.B., Manson, J.E., Stampfer, M.J. *et al.* (2001) Diet, lifestyle and the risk of type 2 diabetes in women. *New England Journal of Medicine* **345**, 790–797.

Iuorno, M.L. & Nestler, J.E. (1999) The polycystic ovary syndrome: treatment with insulin-sensitizing agents. *Diabetes, Obesity Metabolism* 1, 127–136.

James, W.P.T., Astrup, A., Finer, N. *et al.* (2000) Effect of sibutramine on weight maintenance after weight loss: a randomised trial. *Lancet* 356, 2119–2125.

Krentz, A.J. (1999) UKPDS and beyond: into the next millennium. *Diabetes, Obesity and Metabolism* 1, 13–22.

Krentz, A.J. & Bailey C.J. (2001) *Type 2 diabetes in practice.* Royal Society of Medicine Press, London.

Krentz, A.J. & Evans, A. (1998) Selective imidazoline receptor agonists for metabolic syndrome. *Lancet* 351, 152–153.

Krentz, A.J., Ferner, R.E. & Bailey, C.J. (1994) Comparative tolerability profiles of oral antidiabetic agents. *Drug Safety* 11, 223–241.

Lithell, H.O. (1991) Effects of antihypertensive drugs on insulin, glucose and lipid metabolism. *Diabetes Care* 14, 203–209.

Nelson, R.G., Bennett, P.H., Tuomilehto, J., Schersten, B. & Pettitt, D.J. (1995) Preventing non-insulin-dependent diabetes mellitus. *Diabetes* 44, 483–488.

Rendell, M. (2000) Dietary treatment of diabetes mellitus. *New England Journal of Medicine* 342, 1440–1441.

Riddle, M.C. (1998) Learning to use troglitazone. *Diabetes Care* 21, 1389–1391.

Rosenbaum, M. & Leibel, R.L. (1999) The role of leptin in human physiology. *New England Journal of Medicine* 341, 913–915.

Schoonjans, K. & Auwerx, J. (2000) Thiazolidinediones: an update. *Lancet* 355, 1008–1010.

Storlien, L.H., Baur, L.A., Kriketos, A.D. *et al.* (1996) Dietary fats and insulin action. *Diabetologia* 39, 621–631.

Tuomilehto, J., Lindström, J., Eriksson, J.G. *et al.* for the Finnish Diabetes Prevention Study Group (2001) Prevention of type 2 diabetes mellitus by changes in lifestyle among subjects with impaired glucose tolerance. *New England Journal of Medicine* 344, 1343–1350.

UK Prospective Diabetes Study Group. (1998) Intensive blood-glucose control with sulphonylureas or insulin compared with conventional treatment and risk of complications in patients with type 2 diabetes (UKPDS 33). *Lancet* 352, 837–853.

UK Prospective Diabetes Study Group. (1998) Effect of intensive blood-glucose control with metformin on complications in overweight patients with type 2 diabetes (UKPDS 34). *Lancet* 352, 854–865.

UK Prospective Diabetes Study Group. (1998) Tight blood pressure control and risk of macrovascular and microvascular complications in type 2 diabetes (UKPDS 38). *British Medical Journal* 317, 703–713.

UK Prospective Diabetes Study Group. (1998) Efficacy of atenolol and captopril in reducing risk of macrovascular and microvascular complications in type 2 diabetes (UKPDS 39). *British Medical Journal* 317, 713–720.

Wi, M., Gaskill, S.P., Haffner, S.M. & Stern, M.P. (1998) Effects of diabetes and level of glycemia on all-cause and cardiovascular mortality. The San Antonio Heart Study. *Diabetes Care* 21, 1167–1172.

Index

Page numbers in *italics* refer to figures; those in **bold** to tables. Index entries are arranged in letter-by-letter alphabetical order.